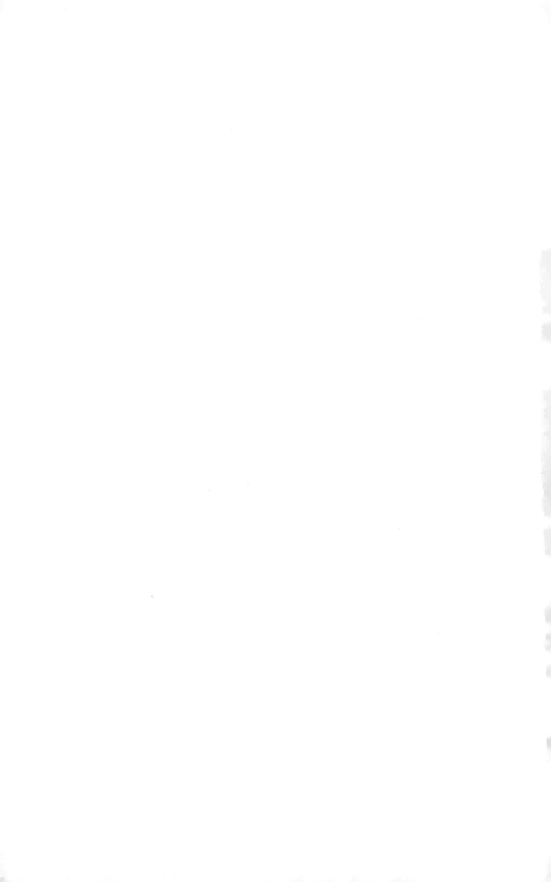

International Perspectives
on Children and Mental Health

INTERNATIONAL PERSPECTIVES ON CHILDREN AND MENTAL HEALTH

Volume 1
Development and Context

Hiram E. Fitzgerald, Kaija Puura,
Mark Tomlinson, and Campbell Paul,
Editors

Child Psychology and Mental Health
Hiram E. Fitzgerald, Series Editor

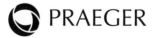 PRAEGER

AN IMPRINT OF ABC-CLIO, LLC
Santa Barbara, California • Denver, Colorado • Oxford, England

Copyright 2011 by ABC-CLIO, LLC

Library of Congress Cataloging-in-Publication Data

International perspectives on children and mental health / Hiram E. Fitzgerald . . . [et al.], editors.
      p. ; cm. — (Child psychology and mental health)
   Includes bibliographical references and indexes.
   ISBN 978-0-313-38298-7 (v.1 : hbk : alk. paper) — ISBN 978-0-313-38299-4 (v.1 : e-ISBN)
1. Child mental health—Cross-cultural studies.   2. Child psychiatry—Cross-cultural
studies.   3. Child development—Cross-cultural studies.   I. Fitzgerald, Hiram E.
II. Series: Child psychology and mental health.
   [DNLM: 1. Child Development.   2. Child.   3. Mental Disorders—prevention &
control.   4. Mental Health. WS 105]
   RJ499.I59   2011
   618.92'89—dc22   2011004642

ISBN: 978-0-313-38298-7
EISBN: 978-0-313-38299-4

15   14   13   12   11   1   2   3   4   5

This book is also available on the World Wide Web as an eBook.
Visit www.abc-clio.com for details.

Praeger
An Imprint of ABC-CLIO, LLC

ABC-CLIO, LLC
130 Cremona Drive, P.O. Box 1911
Santa Barbara, California 93116-1911

This book is printed on acid-free paper (∞)

Manufactured in the United States of America

CONTENTS

SERIES FOREWORD

The 20th century closed with a decade devoted to the study of brain structure, function, and development that, in parallel with studies of the human genome, has revealed the extraordinary plasticity of biobehavioral organization and development. The 21st century opened with a decade focusing on behavior, but the linkages between brain and behavior are as dynamic as the linkages between parents and children and between children and environment.

The Child Psychology and Mental Health series is designed to capture much of this dynamic interplay by advocating for strengthening the science of child development and linking that science to issues related to mental health, child care, parenting, and public policy.

The series consists of individual monographs or thematic volumes, each dealing with a subject that advances knowledge related to the interplay between normal developmental process and developmental psychopathology. The books are intended to reflect the diverse methodologies and content areas encompassed by an age period ranging from conception to late adolescence. Topics of contemporary interest include studies of socioemotional development, behavioral undercontrol, aggression, attachment disorders, substance abuse, and the role that culture and other contextual influences play in shaping developmental trajectories. Investigators involved with prospective longitudinal studies, large epidemiologic cross-sectional samples, or intensely followed clinical cases or those wishing to report a systematic sequence of connected experiments are invited to submit manuscripts. Investigators from all fields in social and behavioral sciences, neurobiological sciences, medical and clinical sciences, and education are invited to submit manuscripts with implications for child and adolescent mental health.

Hiram E. Fitzgerald
Series Editor

PREFACE

In 2002, Praeger Press launched a new series devoted to advancing under-standing of the relationship between child psychology and mental health. The first volume focused on imaginative play in early childhood, and subsequent volumes have examined a wide range of research, policy, and practice issues influencing the mental health of children and adolescents. The collective force of the nine volumes published thus far has provided national stature for the Child Psychology and Mental Health series.

Although population diversity has been represented in past volumes, it has not been a central theme, and therefore past volumes do not provide systematic coverage of the broad issues confronting minority populations. A chapter on juvenile justice disparities among Latino youth, one on tribal boarding schools, and another on the historical impact of slavery on contemporary African American families or the legacy of internment of Japanese families during the Second World War does little justice to the rich set of issues affecting the mental health of children from America's increasingly diverse racioethnic population. Indeed, consensus population estimates indicate that by 2050, at least half of America's children will be members of groups that currently are defined as minorities. The American melting pot is being stirred up, guided by 21st-century recipes that are far more multicultural and inclusive than has been the case in past gen-erations. Despite this unprecedented diversification, little is known about within- and between-group variation in life course pathways for mental health among minority children.

In providing justification for these volumes, I noted that professional and public documents increasingly draw attention to the pervasive problems affecting individual, family, and community development. It was not difficult to point out the extraordinary number of children with poor self-regulatory skills, poor school achievement, and family resources that place them at high risk for achieving successful developmental outcomes. Nor does one have to search hard to find documentation of the long-term effects of child abuse and neglect, gang violence, substance abuse, aggression, poverty, and the dissolution of a sense of community and civic responsibility. All are factors that have fueled a crisis in children's mental health in the United States and throughout the world. In many instances, these issues disproportionately involve children and families of color, exacerbated because of poverty, institutional racism, and a deep sense of anomie. Conversely, in many other families of color, children succeed, families are functioning well, and individual hopes and aspirations are achieved. It is far less common to read about effective parenting, resilience, and life course successes among minority families. Although single volumes have addressed many of these issues, including volumes written by many of the authors attached to the current series, there has been no comprehensive, focused attention directed to articulation of the core issues of child development and mental health within the major minority groups in the United States or internationally.

The time frame from conception to postnatal age five years is vital for all children's development. It is during these years that children develop the neurobiological and social structures that will facilitate brain development and its expression in social-emotional control, self-regulation, literacy and achievement skills, social fitness, health, and well-being. However, while the early years are extraordinarily important in the organization of biopsychosocial regulation, a dynamic and contextual approach to life span development provides ample evidence that there are critical developmental transitions that elementary children, youth, adolescents, and emergent adults must negotiate if they are to construct successful life course pathways. What also is clear is that public access to state-of-the-art knowledge and recommendations about future scientific and public policy practices is limited by a lack of concentrated information about developmental issues facing children and families whose skin color, culture, and racial identities are different from those of children in the dominant population.

This set of nine volumes targets the educated public, individuals who not only are responsible for public policy decisions but also for raising America's children, voting for policy makers, and making decisions about policy issues that may or may not positively affect all children. Two volumes each will address child development and mental health issues in African American children, Latino children, Asian and Pacific Islander children, and children from around the world. One volume covers the same content for American Indian and Alaska Native children. The collective nine volumes capture the state of the art in knowledge known and knowledge to know and examine social and public policies that impede or enhance positive mental health outcomes among an increasingly significant portion of America's children as well as children around the world.

This project would not have been possible without the goodwill and hard work of a dedicated set of editors, uniquely selected for each two-volume set. Their efforts, combined with commitments from an extraordinary group of social, behavioral, and life science scholars, enabled completion within our projected two-year project period. I cannot express deeply enough my thanks to authors for enduring countless e-mail deadline announcements, for their quick responses to tracked-change manuscripts, and for their good spirits throughout the editorial process. Of course, behind the scenes are the individuals who manage the production process. Prior to enrolling in graduate school, Lisa Devereaux provided initial assistance for tracking the flow of editor and author contacts. For most of the duration of the project, Julie Crowgey has served as the project manager, coordinating editors and authors and the publisher to move the project toward its completion. She truly has been the glue that has held everything together. Additional thanks to Adina Huda and Gaukhar Nurseitova for their always perfect and prompt technical assistance with graphics. Finally, I must acknowledge Deborah Carvalko, Praeger editor, who conceived of the idea for the Praeger series and recruited my involvement. It has been a pleasure working with Deborah to produce all the volumes in the Praeger series drawing attention to the interface between child psychology and mental health.

Hiram E. Fitzgerald

Chapter 1

CROOKED TREES GROWING STRAIGHT: THE EXPERIENCES OF BOYS TRANSITIONING OFF THE STREETS OF LA PAZ, BOLIVIA

Kristin Huang and Catherine Ayoub

My father always said I couldn't do anything, that I was a bum, that I was just some street kid. He told me I was never going to study, that I'm just stupid. I wanted to show him that it's not like that. That's why I am studying really hard and trying to do my best in every aspect of my life. . . . You know, the people always say "crooked trees never grow straight." I want to show them that's not true, that people can straighten out, they can get back on the right track and do what they need to do.

—Damian, age 14

The presence of children on the streets is a worldwide phenomenon. Estimates predict there to be up to 170 million street children around the world, with 40 million living in Latin America (United Nations, 1986). Those numbers are increasing daily, primarily due to conflicts and displacement, growing poverty and urban migration, and the spread of HIV (Scanlon, Tomkins, Lynch, & Scanlon, 1998). The problem has reached such proportions that some members of Congress are calling it not just a humanitarian crisis but a security crisis, recommending increased funding to attend to the matter.

Bolivia, the poorest country in South America, is home to its own growing population of street children (Bond, 1993). Approximately 2,500 children are believed to be living on the streets of the three largest cities: La Paz, Cochabamba, and Santa Cruz (UNICEF-Bolivia, 1994). The majority of those children are adolescent boys between 11 and 18 years old (Domic & Ardaya, 1991; UNICEF-Bolivia, 1994). The differences between these children and the many thousands more who are on the streets during the day, but who return home to sleep at night, are slim. Thus the scope of the problem reaches far beyond those sleeping on the streets today and extends to the larger numbers of children considered at risk of sleeping on the streets tomorrow (Scanlon et al., 1998).

The dangers of street life are well documented. Living on the streets puts children at great physical and emotional risk, and the longer children live on the streets, the less likely it is that they will be able to secure a healthy future (Hecht, 1998). There exist no longitudinal studies that offer insight into what happens to children living on the streets in the long run, but common sense indicates that their futures are bleak, if not tragic. Some commit suicide, some are killed as a result of street violence, and others die in tragic accidents related to their vulnerability on the streets. These lost children, along with the others who now roam the streets aimlessly, drooling and unable to talk as a result of their years of constant drug use, make intervention a moral imperative. Though there are various cultural differences among the global population of street children, the lives of those in developing countries have proven to be quite similar in nature (Lalor, 1999; Williams, 1993). Street children in Bolivia, like street children in many other countries, face multiple risks that threaten their development and their lives in general. Lack of adequate shelter, nutrition, education, health care, and loving caretakers puts them at great risk for any number of medical problems, mental illnesses, and social difficulties. The prevalence of drug abuse and unsafe sexual practices among the street children only compounds these risks (Inciardi & Surratt, 1998; Molnar, Shade, Kral, Booth, & Watters, 1998). Preliminary research in La Paz indicates that 89% of street children abuse substances, predominantly inhalants, on a regular basis (Huang, 1998). Studies have also reported that children on the streets become sexually active at a young age, many as young as 10 years old, with few using protection regularly (Anarfi, 1997). As a result, rates of sexually transmitted diseases, unwanted pregnancies, and unsafe abortions are high (Wright, Kaminsky, & Wittig, 1993).

Victimization and exploitation are also part of the daily reality of street life. Studies have shown that most street children are subjected to physical abuse on a regular basis, and many have experienced different forms of sexual abuse as well (Lalor, 1999). Often street children are victimized by other street children, but police are also common perpetrators of physical and sexual violence. It is not unusual for police in Bolivia to round up groups of children arbitrarily, take them to rehabilitation centers, and then beat and rape them (Bond, 1993). In addition, the majority of citizens tend to view street children as nuisances and as little criminals, blaming them for rising crime rates (Ferguson, McIntyre, & Kaminsky, 1993) and sometimes calling for their extermination (Lalor, 1999).

Despite such dangers, children are often reluctant to leave the streets. Practitioners around the world report that helping children transition off the streets and find stability in a residential setting is excruciatingly difficult (Veeran, 2004). Some researchers speculate that drug addiction, lack of trust in adults, and the desire for freedom and independence may be some of the main obstacles preventing children from leaving the streets (Wittig, Wright, & Kaminsky, 1997). Others claim that street children are so focused on the present reality and the need to survive that their ability to consider the long-term risks and consequences of their actions is substantially compromised. These researchers suggest that even when children are able to use such propositional reasoning, their negative outlook on the future affects their ability to care about what may happen as a result of their current decisions (Diversi, Moraes Filho, & Morelli, 1999).

Although the literature on street children offers a compelling call to action as it documents a tragic and worsening reality, it provides limited direction for practitioners. Though the existence of street children and the dangers of street life are well documented, there is a paucity of research related to intervention with this population (Dybicz, 2005) and nothing that specifically addresses how children successfully transition off the streets. In recent years, researchers of runaway and homeless youth in North America began exploring the differences between those who successfully reintegrate into mainstream life and those who remain homeless. Though there are distinct differences between runaway youth in developed countries and street children in developing nations, the specific construct of resilience that emerged from these researchers' efforts provides a useful point of departure for this study.

As Williams, Lindsey, Kurtz, and Jarvis (2001) note, the predominant frameworks in resilience research "do not apply neatly to runaway and homeless youth because such youth frequently are unable or unwilling to alter their exposure to serious risks or successfully engage with caring adults" (p. 235). Furthermore, homeless youth do demonstrate marked resilience as they adapt to life on the streets, creatively utilizing various resources, building supportive social networks, developing their problem-solving skills, and honing an ability to discern who is trustworthy (Bender, Thompson, McManus, Lantry, & Flynn, 2007; Kidd & Davidson, 2007). To improve intervention efforts, therefore, it is necessary to distinguish the resilience of successfully reintegrated runaway youth from general concepts of resilience. The small body of research dedicated to this specific task separates resilience into three central categories: personal attributes, critical incidents, and resources.

Several personal attributes distinguish youth who have been able to transition off the streets. Determination is a primary attribute that appears throughout the literature (Kidd & Davidson, 2007; Lindsey, Kurtz, Jarvis, Williams, & Nackerud, 2000). Youth who have successfully left the streets frequently demonstrate tenacity and persistence and possess what Williams et al. (2001, p. 242) call that "I'll show you!" attitude. This attribute is often accompanied by pride in overcoming adversity (Kidd & Davidson, 2007; Williams et al., 2001). Those youth who are able to derive a sense of personal value or self-esteem from having survived adverse circumstances are more likely to succeed in leaving the streets, believing they are capable of something better (Kidd & Davidson, 2007; Lindsey et al., 2000).

Spirituality is another primary attribute of resilient runaway youth. The ability to find meaning and purpose in life experiences as well as draw on a higher power for strength and comfort seems to be critical for many youth making the transition off the streets (Bender et al., 2007; Williams et al., 2001). This seems particularly relevant in light of Rew, Taylor-Seehafer, Thomas, and Yockey's (2001) study, which found that hopelessness and connectedness explained 50% of the variance in resilience in homeless adolescents.

Finally, resilient runaway youth demonstrate an ability to learn from difficult experiences, developing new attitudes and behaviors that facilitate the transition off the streets (Lindsey et al., 2000). Critical among those new attitudes is the readiness to accept help (Bender et al., 2007; Williams et al., 2001) that often follows critical incidents (MacKnee & Mervyn, 2002).

Though the path off the streets is different for each youth, critical incidents can play a key role in propelling that path forward. For some youth, the transition off the streets is more sudden, often following a wake-up call experience, whereas for others, it is a more gradual process, "characterized by cycles of progress and regress" (Lindsey et al., 2000, p. 138). In a 2002 study, MacKnee and Mervyn identified 19 different critical incidents that facilitated homeless people's transition off the streets. They organized the incidents across five central themes that included (1) establishing supportive relationships, (2) discovering some measure of self-esteem, (3) accepting personal responsibilities, (4) accomplishing mainstream lifestyle goals, and (5) changing perceptions. Significant events that have been shown to activate these themes include reconnecting with supportive family members, completing a degree program, having a near-death experience or losing someone close, having the opportunity to help someone else, having responsibility for a pet, and feeling like you have hit bottom (Bender et al., 2007; Kurtz, Lindsey, Jarvis, & Nackerud, 2000; Lindsey et al., 2000; MacKnee & Mervyn, 2002; Williams et al., 2001).

Resources in conjunction with critical incidents facilitate a transition off the streets. Since critical incidents can frequently lead to an increased readiness to accept help (MacKnee & Mervyn, 2002; Williams et al., 2001), the presence of key resources during or immediately after significant incidents is advantageous (Kurtz et al., 2000). Key resources in helping youth transition off the streets are primarily human resources (Bender et al., 2007; Kurtz et al., 2000; Lindsey et al., 2000). Family, friends, and professional helpers represent the main human resources that provide assistance to youth on the streets, and they have the potential both to help and to hinder resilience (Kidd & Davidson, 2007; Kurtz et al., 2000). According to street youth, the types of help that are most important are caring, trustworthiness, setting boundaries and holding youth accountable, concrete assistance, and professional counseling (Kurtz et al., 2000). Help that is long-term and consistent (Williams et al., 2001), flexible and person centered, and that can productively engage family members and friends in supportive roles (Kurtz et al., 2000) is thought to best promote resilience and help youth make the transition off the streets.

Social scientists and practitioners agree that more research is needed to illuminate the experiences of street children (Hutz & Koller, 1999). Earls and Carlson (1999) discuss the need for "nuanced research" and advocate for the use of qualitative methods to "provide complex and intimate depictions of the relationships and difficulties of the children's experience" (p. 78). In response to this call, our study aims to provide a starting point for practice-focused research by exploring the journeys of boys who were able to leave the streets successfully. Its goals are to capture the lived experiences of these boys as they moved onto and off of the streets and to develop an understanding of what the boys believe enabled their transition success. The questions guiding this project are as follows:

1. How do the boys describe their lives prior to moving to the streets?
2. How do they describe the process of transitioning onto the streets?
3. How did they view their lives on the streets?
4. How do they describe the process of leaving the streets?
5. What did the process of becoming stabilized in a residential program involve?
6. What do they believe enabled their transition success?

ETHNOGRAPHIC APPROACHES TO
UNDERSTANDING BOLIVIAN BOYS
ON THE STREET

Because the population we wished to study comprises extremely vulnerable children, and because access to that population is complicated, sample choices were made in an effort to minimize risk and maximize resources. Consequently, we selected 10 children currently living in the Esperanza permanent homes; the names of the homes have been changed to protect the identities of participants. While using such a sample of convenience has obvious drawbacks, it provided a reasonable and feasible way to proceed.

The 10 children living in the Esperanza permanent homes are boys between the ages of 13 and 17 who have successfully transitioned off the streets. Boys are considered "successfully transitioned" after demonstrating a minimum of nine months of stability in a transition home, characterized by no running away, no drug use, and a willingness and ability to participate in all program activities. All 10 boys graduated from the Esperanza transition program within the past four years, spent a minimum of one year on the streets prior to coming into the program, and experienced some degree of abuse and neglect in their original families. According to local reconnaissance, these boys are representative of the larger population of boys living on the streets of La Paz (UNICEF-Bolivia, 1994).

The boys are all residents in permanent homes run by the Esperanza Program, a U.S.-based nonprofit organization that supports and runs programs to address the needs of street children in La Paz, Bolivia. The Esperanza Program offers three different types of direct-service programs that are interconnected and successive. The first is the street outreach program, through which outreach workers identify and build relationships with children living on the streets, with the primary objective of helping them decide to enter the second program: the transition home. Though street outreach activities are open to anyone, the program currently only targets boys between the ages of 6 and 13 for entry into its residential program. Street outreach services include basic medical care and health education, regular social and recreational activities, advocacy, and friendly support visits to check in on children.

All the participants came into the transition home through the street outreach program. The transition home offers a highly structured program that includes psychoeducational groups, remedial education, and various extracurricular activities, all focused on helping the boys adapt to life off the streets. Once boys reach a level of stability, typically 9–15 months later, they are able to move to a permanent home. Esperanza's permanent homes utilize a family model in which 10 boys and a set of house parents live together in a house. Boys continue to receive various support services, but they attend public school and enjoy more freedoms as they grow in their stability. Boys remain in the permanent homes until adulthood; as adults, they are encouraged to return to the home and to consider the members of the home their families. The program has no fixed age limit; rather it plans to base decisions regarding the transition to independence on the individual needs of each boy.

The general structure of the Esperanza residential program is one that is used by multiple programs in Bolivia. Many residential programs engage in street outreach activities to form initial relationships with children, run transition houses for children first coming off the streets, and then move children into more permanent living situations once they have demonstrated stability. Therefore an examination of how children who progressed through this type of residential program experienced the transition process bears direct implications for a large community of programs. Since residential programs are the primary vehicle through which children in La Paz achieve stability off the streets, it makes sense to examine children's transition experiences in a context that includes residential living. This approach also allows us to offer suggestions to enhance success of residential programs for homeless youth.

ANALYSIS OF NARRATIVES FROM BOYS OF THE STREET

In keeping with the approach recommended by Earls and Carlson (1999), qualitative methods were selected for use in this study in order to respond to research questions that address process, context, and meaning. Since such an approach is more likely to "offer insight, enhance understanding, and provide a meaningful guide to action," it was considered appropriate, given the research goals (Strauss & Corbin, 1998, p. 12). The primary methods used to collect data were individual interviews and focus groups. All interviews and focus groups were conducted by one researcher in Spanish, tape-recorded, and then transcribed verbatim for analysis.

Whereas in-depth individual interviews explored the perspectives and experiences of each boy independently, focus groups provided the additional benefit of stimulating the participants to "think beyond their own private thoughts and to articulate their opinions" (Kleiber, 2004, p. 91). The authors anticipated that the adolescent boys might have difficulty elaborating on their thoughts and reflecting deeply on the questions posed in a one-on-one session without significant prompting from the facilitator. Focus groups were therefore implemented as an additional data collection method because of their distinct methodological advantages for research with children and adolescents, in particular, since they tend to facilitate participation and more clearly elicit perceptions and beliefs (Vaughn, Schumm, & Sinagub, 1996). Using individual interviews and focus groups together allowed for a more comprehensive sense of the boys' transition experiences and provided multiple opportunities to triangulate information.

Each boy participated in an initial focus group and two individual, semi-structured interviews on separate occasions during a two-week period. Each interview lasted between 35 and 60 minutes. The first interview focused on their life experiences from birth through their time on the streets, whereas the second focused on their experiences from the streets to the present. Though the interviewer had an interview protocol as a guide, participants were encouraged simply to tell their life stories.

The follow-up focus groups were conducted a few months after the interviews and were led like brainstorming sessions. Participants were asked to make meaning of several scenarios and respond to questions, not personally, but as if they were speaking for the general population of boys in a similar position to theirs. In general, reflection on meaning did not come easily to participants, and a certain amount of probing was necessary to solicit deeper personal analysis. In the end, the data collected through both individual interviews and focus groups converged on similar themes that reflected the opinions of the boys.

A grounded theory approach to analysis was taken in order to allow the data to drive theory development (Strauss & Corbin, 1998). Preconceived lists of concepts and themes were eschewed as much as possible in favor of an open coding process (Strauss & Corbin, 1998). The software program NVivo was used to store, organize and analyze data.

After each interview and focus group was transcribed, each transcript was coded twice. The first coding pass attempted to establish a general chronology of events, as well as to document background information. This supported the construction of a general framework of each child's transition process as it related to time and place and significant event. After reviewing each case for these details, we used data matrices (Miles & Huberman, 1994) to organize initial findings and compare the general transition process across cases. Findings continuously informed the data collection process and analytic memos were written to document emerging theories and their influence on any changes in methods.

In the second analysis, more abstract concepts were examined. Both categorizing and contextualizing strategies were used to organize the data and build theory. Emerging themes and patterns were identified, using "in vivo" codes as appropriate to preserve the cultural context of the data. This was followed by the categorization of data within and across each case according to prominent themes related to the research questions. All data was reviewed periodically in light of developing theories, following the grounded theory approach.

DESCRIPTION OF THE BOYS AND THEIR
LIFE TRAJECTORIES

The 10 adolescent boys ranged in age from 13 to 17 and were homeless for between one and five years prior to entering the program. The boys' residency in Esperanza's permanent homes meant that they had successfully transitioned off of the streets and achieved stability in a transition home, earning the move to a permanent residential facility. Half of the boys lived in Hogar Illimani (Illimani Home) and the other half lived in Hogar Sajama (Sajama Home). While the boys of Hogar Illimani were generally older and had been off the streets longer, all of the boys had been off the streets for a minimum of about two years at the time of the interviews (see Table 1.1).

While it was difficult for the boys to provide precise information with regard to time and place, it was possible to get a general sense of their paths from their original homes to their current homes. All of the boys reported spending increasing amounts of time on the streets from the time they were very young. All but one began sleeping on the streets when they were between seven and nine years old. The length of time between when participants first left home and when they entered the Esperanza Program ranged from one to five years, although it is unclear precisely what amount of this time was spent living on the streets, since eight participants spent time in other institutions and several reported movement to and from their family homes. This movement back and forth, however, tended to be during the beginning of the boys' time on the streets and diminished over time.

On the streets, the boys slept in various places and roamed about during waking hours looking for money. Some lived in an abandoned factory building with a group of boys, others lived in makeshift shelters alongside the sewer, and a few slept in trees. All earned money through stealing, though some also begged or had jobs. Working as a *voceador*, shouting destinations out of the window of busses, was the most common job held

Table 1.1
Participant profiles

	Martin	Lucho	Franklin	Diego	Damian	Florentino	Adrian	Alex	Tito	Cristian
DOB	10-8-92	9-12-89	11-4-89	1-2-90	8-11-92	9-5-92	3-31-93	3-5-91	12-23-93	12-6-89
Home	Sajama	Illimani	Illimani	Illimani	Illimani	Sajama	Sajama	Sajama	Sajama	Illimani
Age (at time of interview)	14	17	17	17	14	14	14	15	13	17
Age when entered home	12	10	12	13	10	12	12	13	11	12
Length of time off streets	1 year 11 months	6 years 7 months	5 years 4 months	4 years 7 months	4 years 2 months	2 years 3 months	1 year 10 months	1 year 11 months	2 years 2 months	5 years 7 months
Age first living on streets	7	7	11	9	7	9	7	9	9	9
Length of time homeless[a]	5 years	2–3 years	1 year	3 years	3 years	3 years	5 years	4 years	2 years	2 years
Experience in other institutions	Yes	Yes	No	?	Yes	Yes	Yes	Yes	Yes	Yes
Drug Use	Tried it	None	None	?	Tried it	Habitual user	Habitual user	Habitual user	Habitual user	Tried it
School attendance while on streets	Dropped out	Dropped out	Dropped out	Dropped out	Stayed in school	Dropped out	Dropped out	Dropped out	Dropped out	Dropped out
How connected to program	Through street outreach	Through street outreach	Through street outreach	Through street outreach	Through street outreach	Through street outreach	Through street outreach	Through street outreach	Through street outreach	Through street outreach

[a]This number reflects the length of time between when participants started living on the streets and when they entered their current residential programs. During this time, most participants had stints in other institutions, and in some cases, participants returned home for brief periods.

by the boys, though some also worked washing dishes or preparing foods during street festivals. Most of the boys had experience inhaling paint thinner, though only four admitted to being habitual users. All but one of the participants dropped out of school when they left home and did not receive formal schooling again until they entered the permanent homes of Esperanza.

All of the boys became connected with the Esperanza Program through the program's street outreach workers. Some participated in outreach activities (soccer games, special holiday events, medical care) and built relationships with staff members over time, while others met staff members during times when they made street visits. One boy came to know staff members through a hospital referral when he was receiving inpatient care for a street-related health problem.

FROM HOME TO THE STREET: FAMILY BACKGROUNDS

All 10 participants were born and raised in the greater La Paz area. While some spent time living in the country and jungle regions just outside of the metropolitan area, they all were raised primarily in the city of La Paz or in the slum suburb of El Alto. All participants were of indigenous or mixed descent and came from impoverished backgrounds. Their homes were simple and sometimes quite rustic. As Adrian described, "My family had few resources, just like any other. We had a bed, a stove, that's it." Some referred to their homes as "a room," others talked about needing to fetch water. Damian described his first home saying, "There wasn't water, there wasn't light. We had to use candles and for water we had to go to the plaza . . . and bring it all the way up the hill." Despite the humble nature of his home, Tito said, "To me it was nice." All of the boys' families struggled to make ends meet. Their caregivers found employment mainly in service positions, hard labor, or selling food on the streets; periods of unemployment were not uncommon.

Participants came from different family constellations (see Table 1.2). Some had large families with multiple half siblings, others had smaller families with fewer children, and two were raised by relatives surrounded by various cousins. Only three boys had relationships with their fathers, and six were raised primarily by single women. Three of the boys lost their mothers at an early age; two were subsequently raised by their fathers and the other was raised by his grandmother.

Lucho never knew either of his parents and was raised by an aunt. Martin didn't know who his real family was, but lived with a few different

Table 1.2
Family backgrounds

	Martin	Lucho	Franklin	Diego	Damian	Florentino	Adrian	Alex	Tito	Cristian
Primary caregiver(s)	Unclear	Aunt	Mother, then father and stepmother	Both parents, then father	Both parents	Mother, grandparents	Mother	Mother	Both parents, then mother	Grandmother
Other children in the family	Unclear	Various cousins	Younger brother, half brothers	Older brother, various older half siblings	Older twin siblings who died, younger sisters	Older sisters	Various half siblings	Various half siblings	Older sister	Various cousins
Caregiver employment	Unclear	Washing clothes	Caretaker, masonry	Mining, carpentry, washing clothes, selling food	Odd jobs, selling food on street	Made and sold cheese	Selling candy on street	Sweeping streets	Secretarial work (?), building roads	Looked for work on the street
Physical abuse	Yes	Yes	None reported	Yes	Yes	Yes	Yes	None reported[a]	Yes	Yes
Neglect[b]	Yes	Yes	Yes	Yes	Yes	None reported	None reported	None reported	None reported	None reported
Domestic violence	Yes	None reported	Yes	Yes	Yes	None reported	None reported	None reported	Yes	None reported
Abandonment or loss	Unclear who real family is	Both parents died	Mother murdered when he was 7 or 8	Mother died of unknown illness/injury	Twin siblings died of illness	Father never present	Father never present	Father never present	Father left when he was around 3 or 4	Mother died giving birth to younger sibling (who also died), father left

[a] Alex reported extreme forms of physical abuse inflicted on his older siblings but never reported experiencing physical abuse himself.

[b] Neglect is only indicated in cases where the participant reported feeling either emotionally or physically neglected.

substitute families and their extended relatives through what seemed to be informal arrangements. Damian was the only participant who had a relationship with both parents at the time he left home, though they were separated at the time. Despite the differences in makeup, all the families could be described as broken. Whether through abandonment, loss, or divorce, all of the families were torn apart. Those that started out intact experienced domestic violence and ultimately, separation.

LIFE WITH THEIR FAMILIES OF ORIGIN

Words like "fine," "OK," and "good," were the first to come up when most participants began describing life in their original homes. However, the details that followed these initial adjectives were predominantly negative. Physical abuse, neglect, abandonment, loss, and domestic violence were key themes that came out of the boys' narratives of their prestreet years. Though not all of the boys experienced all of those kinds of traumas, most experienced more than one and nearly all experienced physical abuse and some form of loss or abandonment.

Though Martin was the only boy to speak of physical neglect, emotional neglect was discussed by several of the boys. Damian described neglect as feeling "disappointed" and "unloved." Diego, who lived with his father after his mother's death, described a lack of positive attention. "[My father] would just come home saying, 'I want something to eat.' I knew how to cook so I would cook for him. But I don't know, I just felt like I didn't have any kind of support in school, all of that. He didn't have any kind of discipline." Diego resented the fact that his father did not notice him and would just use him as a cook. He yearned for someone to give him boundaries, to reign in his misbehavior and make sure he was going to school. Instead, his father hardly noticed when Diego started skipping school, and when he did find out, he did not do anything about it.

Lack of involvement and supervision was not uncommon. Caregivers were often gone for long periods of time working. Sometimes, like in Franklin's case, a caregiver would travel to another city for work, leaving the children home alone and unattended for days or weeks at a time. More often caregivers would leave children alone all day and into the evening while they worked or tried to find work. It was easy, then, to run to the streets and there was great incentive to do so.

SCHOOL EXPERIENCES

All of the boys attended public schools in La Paz or in the suburb of El Alto prior to living on the street. State-run schools (*colegios fiscales*) offer three sessions of classes each day, so boys attended school either in the morning, the afternoon or the evening for about three to four hours a day. All but one of the boys described school in neutral or negative terms. Adrian had nothing negative to say about his school experience but dropped out after the third grade. Cristian said school was "fine" but that he did not really have any friends. Diego had a similar experience and frequently chose to spend time on the streets in lieu of going to school. Franklin had a distinctly negative school experience, describing it as "terrible! There were these bullies and this one guy always bothered me and wanted to fight with me. I didn't want to go back there because there were always problems, fights, all of that."

Damian was the only boy who talked about a positive school experience and was the only 1 of the 10 not to drop out of school during the time he was on the streets. Damian's relationship with a particular teacher had a profound effect on his commitment to education. When Damian's family situation deteriorated and he left home for the streets, he continued attending school and made sure he was enrolled each year. Bolivian schools require students to have a *libreta*, a formal document that verifies their school record, in order to enroll and attend school each year. While on the streets, Damian carried his *libreta* in his backpack wherever he went and took great care not to lose it. He said that he learned in school that studying was the way to "a happy life," so he was committed to graduating. During the time of his interview, he was on track to finish high school at 17, a fact he readily shared.

RUNNING FROM HOME TO THE STREETS

The transition onto the streets was, in most cases, the result of a combination of factors. Some of those factors, like abuse, neglect and domestic violence pushed participants out of their homes and onto the streets. Other factors, like arcades, opportunities to socialize with other kids, and money-making opportunities, were persistent temptations that pulled them onto the streets. In general, whether participants were primarily running *from* their homes or running *to* the streets, the street ultimately was deemed a better alternative to their homes.

For a few participants, the move to the streets was more sudden and definitive. Cristian, after experiencing a harsh beating from his grandfather that left a scar, ran away and never looked back. "I was so furious I just left," he explained, and out of fear he never returned. Lucho, who was spending more and more time on the streets, returned home late one night and was punished by his aunt. He spent a month confined to his room and finally decided he had had enough and left. When he heard his aunt was looking for him, he took care to hide. "I was afraid she would punish me, or that I would be left alone. I never wanted to be like that again," he commented. Though Tito was accustomed to spending long days and evenings on the streets, he also left home abruptly. Like Cristian, Tito claimed it was an abusive incident that precipitated his departure. For most participants, however, the move to the streets was more gradual. A growing discontentment in their homes led to more and more time on the streets during the day, followed by stints of time staying out all night or sleeping in other places.

THE MEANING OF STREET LIFE

For all of the boys, living on the streets was a preferential option over staying in their homes. Many of the boys saw their lives on the streets as "free" and without hassles. Florentino did not see a big distinction between his home life and his street life. He explained, "It was practically like living in my house. When I lived at home, I could go wherever but I had to ask permission. On the streets, I went where I wanted when I wanted."

Though freedom was a ubiquitous theme throughout the boys' stories of their lives on the streets, themes of shame and sadness were also present. Several boys talked about the negative ways in which they were viewed by others. They often felt embarrassed by their appearance and by the fact that they were homeless. According to Diego, "People looked at you bad. I didn't like for people to see me in the streets." Martin said living on the streets meant he "didn't exist in the world, because people didn't see me as a good kid. They just saw me as a street kid who robbed and did bad things." Like Martin, Tito disliked people's perception of him as bad. "No one treats you well," he said, "They see you coming and they get scared, thinking you're gonna do something to them." Many boys felt similarly misunderstood and talked about how others saw them as worthless.

Most of the boys expressed negative self-perceptions when discussing their time on the streets and were aware, at least on some level, that street life had a down side. Tito said, "I was nothing, I was just a bum." Martin was aware that living on the streets had negative implications for his future, but he struggled with *vicios* (vices). He explained, "I knew [living on the streets] meant I wasn't going to be able to do anything. . . . But the streets were always chasing me." This kind of awareness was not claimed by all of the boys. Adrian admitted he never thought about the significance of living in the streets. "I just wanted to be the way I was."

Cristian explained that "when you are on the streets you forget about everything. You forget what day it is because all the days are the same," admitting that he, too, did not give the consequences of street life much thought. Damian, however, said it was hard not to be aware of the dangers of street life. "I knew that it was ruining me. Because I knew several kids who were just totally messed up. You could see it."

TRANSITIONING: DECIDING TO LEAVE THE STREETS

The first part of the boys' transition experiences involved making the decision to leave the streets. There were three main reasons the boys gave for making this decision: real and present dangers, wanting to change, and nothing to lose. Like with their transitions onto the streets, both push and pull factors contributed to the boys' decision making.

For some of the boys, dangers and threats on the streets pushed them to decide to leave. In Cristian's case, that threat was an older street boy named Jaime, who made Cristian his "slave" and threatened his life. Cristian saw an opportunity to enter a residential program as a way to get away from Jaime and avoid the violence he was sure to inflict. For other boys, fear of police brutality was a motivating force. Thus for these boys, deciding to leave the streets was about self-protection and escape from danger.

For several other boys, deciding to leave the streets was about wanting to change their lives. They were drawn off of the streets by the promise of something better. Adrian feared what he would become if he stayed on the streets. "I was afraid I would be Mr. Nobody! I was thinking I would just be like some bum, so I was thinking I have to study and become someone in life." To him, entering a home was an opportunity to become educated and find a real identity. Alex started thinking about changing his life after a visit from his mother. Alex was motivated by both his mother's emotional disappointment and a feeling that he was losing himself to the streets. He perceived a distinct point of no return on the streets; he wanted to change his life before it was too late.

Damian knew that leaving the streets was the only way he could change his life. According to him, "On the streets, there are different choices or paths, let's say, and the majority of them lead to throwing your life away. There is only one that doesn't and for me that is leaving the streets, abstaining, changing." During his time on the streets, he had a nagging desire to change his life. "I don't know how to say it," he explained, "but it was like something ticking inside of me, telling me that I'm not that kind of person, that I can get out of all this." His decision to change his life by entering a home was influenced by a strong desire to demonstrate that he could "be better."

For a few of the boys, deciding to leave the streets and enter a home was neither about escaping dangers nor making life changes. When the opportunity came along to go with street outreach workers to the Esperanza Program's transition home, they figured they would give it a try because they had nothing to lose. It was only after leaving the streets and entering Esperanza's transition home that Diego and the other boys with nothing to lose made more conscious decisions to truly leave street life.

TRANSITIONING: COMING OFF THE STREETS

From the perspective of the boys, transition off the streets was primarily about changing their lives. This section documents how they characterized the changes that occurred during the process of becoming stabilized in a permanent home. The changes the boys described were personal, internal changes. The examples they offered could be divided into five main categories: behavioral, emotional/relational, spiritual, cognitive, and identity.

For all the boys, changes in their behavior were a big part of their transition process. Leaving the streets and entering a home required them to give up certain behaviors and adopt new ones that were less familiar. For several of the boys, stealing and inhaling paint thinner were intense addictions. Giving up those *vicios* required no small amount of effort. The boys were unable to describe what it was like to overcome those addictions, but they counted their success in doing so among their biggest achievements. Adrian said he knew he had successfully transitioned because "I don't think about drugs anymore. I don't think about stealing."

Learning to treat others with respect was a change many boys considered a big part of their transition process. Tito described himself before he entered the transition home as "a punk." "I didn't respect other people," he said, "but I've been improving." One of the main ways in which Alex changed, he said, is that "I don't swear much anymore or say rude things. . . . Like I don't want to say those words, like fu . . . or sh . . . right? Because when I started school again, I didn't talk like that anymore and it felt different." Talking with respect made him feel like a different person, and the difference felt good.

A few boys discussed powerful emotional changes that took place during their transition process that also helped them develop better relationships with others. Franklin described himself prior to entering the Esperanza homes as "a loner, very closed off." He struggled to relate to others and had mostly superficial relationships as a result. He cited "changing in my ability to socialize with others" as one of the biggest changes he experienced in transitioning off of the streets, crediting staff members with helping him become "more open." Franklin also talked about a second change, learning to manage his emotions. Lucho talked about learning how to trust as a major emotional change he experienced. After stabilizing in a permanent home, he "felt more trusting, more secure." The relationships he developed as a result made him feel "like I had my own home."

Spiritual change was another way the transition process was characterized. Several boys attributed their transition success to spiritual changes that occurred during the transition process. For example, Cristian reported that he was more open to receiving help from his counselors after he connected with a higher power. He was more willing to accept their authority and follow rules when he felt something larger was a stake. He seemed comfortable with the idea of submitting to God's authority, but less comfortable with the idea of doing something simply because a counselor said so. Thus, connecting with a higher power made him open to the assistance counselors had to offer and he was able to attend to the problems in his life with greater seriousness. For Martin, transition was about realizing that continuous growth is a vital part of existence. Developing a spiritual life helped him to commit to working hard and learning, by helping him redefine life as a growth process. This gave his life a distinct future orientation, which was not as present when he was on the streets.

Many of the boys also spoke about developing new perspectives as part of their transition process. Transitioning, according to the boys, was learning to see street life as dangerous and the pleasures it offered as only temporary. This cognitive shift was a central part of the change they experienced in becoming stable in a permanent home. In the process of transitioning, Martin came to the realization that "having things" was not going to make him "somebody." He learned that education had more redeeming value over "things" and set about redefining himself as a student instead of a street kid. Franklin had trouble accepting the rules of the Esperanza homes at first and sometimes missed the freedom of the streets. Part of his transition process was recognizing that it was in his interest to put up with them. He also became more conscious of his actions and what he could accomplish with a little foresight. "Before," he explained, "I did whatever I had to do, but never with any sense of purpose. Now I've learned that you need to plan things."

Self-redefinition was the final change reported by the boys. For many, change was about "becoming somebody," leaving behind their previous identities as "punks," "bums," and "nothings." For most, that happened through education. "[Studying] to become a professional was my only desire when I came here," explained Florentino, "I want[ed] to be someone in life." His commitment to this new identity helped him stay on track and resist temptations. When family members visited him in the transition home and offered to buy him various things if he returned home, he decided against the offer because he knew if he stayed, he might be able to make up a year of school that he lost. "I didn't want all those things," he explained, "I didn't care if they bought me anything or not. That used to be important to me, but now it's all about studying, not the streets and all that." Though many of the boys felt they had left their previous "street kid" identities behind as they made the transition off of the streets, several were still working toward "becoming someone" and believed that goal would be fulfilled when they graduated and "became professionals." Thus, identity change was not simply binary but was seen as an evolving process.

PERCEPTIONS AND INFLUENCE OF THE
ESPERANZA RESIDENTIAL PROGRAM

In the boys' narratives of their experiences transitioning off of the streets they described their ability to successfully stabilize in the Esperanza Program. When reflecting on what enabled them to stay in Esperanza's transition homes, many boys first referenced their experiences in other homes to explain what was different this time. These experiences influenced their perception of Esperanza, which was directly related to their decisions to stay in the program and not run back to the streets again. All but two of the boys reported that they spent time living in other residential programs prior to entering Esperanza; most had lived in four or more. In general, the boys described their experiences in other homes negatively, which is not surprising given their departure from each one. The most frequent complaint proffered was abuse from older boys. According to several boys, other homes were crowded and overrun with kids and the quality of care provided was lacking.

Some programs required the boys to work selling things during the day to earn money to support their own care. Cristian failed to see how that was helpful. "Since I knew how to steal, that was easier and faster," he admitted. Other homes offered programming or structures that some boys found helpful, but allowed boys to be on the streets during the day which ultimately undermined those efforts. Tito particularly liked one program's evening classes and tiered structure. He initially did well there and worked his way up to the second highest level, enjoying the better quality rooms and privileges. But since he spent a good portion of each day with friends on the street, he eventually fell back into using drugs, lost his privileged status, and left the home.

For some of the boys, Esperanza was just another program. They were not drawn to it for any particular reason, but when they had the opportunity to visit, they opted to see if it suited them. In these cases, the nature of the program had no impact on the boys' decision to leave the streets. For other boys, however, the program as it was presented to the boys by street outreach workers, did have particular appeal. Adrian, who was in the hospital recovering from a street-related illness, was planning to return to the streets upon his release but was intrigued by an outreach worker's description of the program. "[She said] it's for 10 boys and after you are rehabilitated, you can go to another house where you have a mom and a dad. That sounded good to me because on the streets you don't have a mom and dad." Other boys were not aware of program specifics until after they arrived at the transition home, but also mentioned the "family-like" atmosphere as a key part of their attraction to the program. Franklin admitted he never tried another home because he had been discouraged by the descriptions his street friends provided and followed their advice to "not bother." But Esperanza seemed "different," he said, "I felt accompanied by the counselors and other boys, like it was a family, together and not alone."

The boys identified various resources, experiences, and supports at the Esperanza houses that helped them make a successful transition off of the streets. Their accounts of helpful intervention fell into four general categories: human and spiritual support, programmatic support, getting an education, and focusing on the future.

The boys talked about human supports that they found especially helpful. For many boys, human support was about having adults they could "go to with problems" who would respond with help. Tito said he feels "happy" because he has people who "understand and listen" to him. The advice and encouragement offered by adults (primarily their counselors), particularly during intense periods, made a substantial difference in the boys' ability to achieve stability. During their time in the transition home, most boys struggled with the temptation to run back to the streets. Running tended to be their default reaction to conflict or stress during the early stages of the transition process until they developed other methods of conflict resolution. Martin claimed that in those difficult moments, "everyone helped me. They would say 'Don't go. Think about it.' They would make me wait an hour . . . so I would think and reflect and then I would stay."

Like Martin, Tito benefited from taking time to carefully think through his decisions. He also saw counselors use their own advice, which helped him trust its value. He took notice of how the counselors were able to cope with their own life challenges and still interact in positive and supportive ways with him and the other boys in the home. That they did not take their anger out on him when they arrived went against his previous experience and stood as a living lesson in anger management. Other boys mentioned that talking with counselors helped them feel "a lot calmer" and "less depressed," and that the help they offered made them feel "supported" and "cared for."

The experience of being trusted by counselors was another way in which the boys felt supported. For a few boys, the chore of buying bread at the local bakery meant far more than coming home with breakfast. It was a test of their trustworthiness and a measure of their transition progress. For Florentino, it was when he was asked to buy bread that he began to realize he had changed. "They started trusting me," he explained with pride, "First they would give us like 20 pesos to go buy bread in the morning. Sometimes they sent me with even 100 pesos. It made me feel happy."

In addition to counselors and house parents, family members also served as key supports for some boys. It was unclear how many of the boys had contact with family members during their transition process and to what extent, but several mentioned that having their residency in the home endorsed by members of their family had a significant impact on their ability to stay. Florentino appreciated his family's support. His sister's characterization of the home as a fortunate opportunity helped Florentino see more clearly the advantages he would have if he stayed. He was inspired to not repeat his sister's mistakes.

Many of the boys cited the spiritual support and moral teaching they received as instrumental in helping them make the transition off of the streets. The lessons they learned through formal and informal instruction, and through individual reflection helped them make the changes they deemed necessary for successful transition. One of the primary instructional vehicles mentioned as helpful by the boys were "devotionals." Alex credits the devotionals with helping him learn "to recognize my mistakes, that nobody is perfect, that we're always going to make mistakes. Even grown ups make mistakes, too." For Alex, the devotionals fine-tuned his sense of right and wrong, which improved his ability to assess his own behavior and make better choices. The message that "it's OK to make mistakes" was the preeminent lesson he learned, suggesting that perhaps forgiveness was of some importance in his transition experience.

In addition, boys learned and were taught things they considered valuable through group counseling sessions, informal conversations with caregivers, and opportunities for personal reflection. They learned about "what is good and what is bad," how their actions affect others, and how far they have come, all of which helped them develop stability off of the streets. The group counseling sessions taught Alex "that we have to respect each other . . . that we don't have to fight, that we can talk to each other in a nice manner." Tito considered learning how to respect others particularly important, too, "because if you don't respect someone, they are not going to respect you. They told us that respect breeds respect." As they learned to "talk with respect" and rely less on physical aggression, they saw the benefits of this wisdom.

Informal conversations with caregivers reinforced the lessons taught in more formal instructional settings and helped the boys examine certain behaviors with increased perspective. Martin said talking with counselors, "helped me realize that when you steal money from a woman or a man, you leave them without anything. . . . When I was in the street, I didn't really care if I hurt people. I didn't even know if I hurt them or not."

Many of the boys also mentioned certain programmatic supports that included consistent structure, boundaries and responsibilities. Lucho appreciated the full daily routine. He liked having a sense of purpose from the moment he woke up in the morning and felt good being productive. Florentino liked having a schedule, as well, and added that "It helps because . . . like if I'm going to play soccer for an hour and then do my homework for an hour, that's my plan. If I don't have that schedule, then I'd play soccer for two hours and I wouldn't have time to do my homework." Having a structured schedule to which he was held accountable helped him manage his time and accomplish daily goals that he otherwise might not have accomplished. Tito appreciated the value of having responsibilities. Through chores like washing his clothes, Tito was able to see the value of his own work. The effort he put in would be reflected in his appearance and that motivated him to do a good job. Thus, having responsibilities helped him develop a work ethic, and having a work ethic helped define him as something other than a bum.

Social activities were also frequently mentioned for their value in the transition process. Florentino said that "spending time with the other boys and counselors, playing, at lunch, joking around" was what really helped him to adapt to life off the streets. This answer was curious since he had also mentioned spending time with his family when he lived at home. He explained the difference saying, "I hung out with my family, but I didn't really know them. And sometimes you get bored when every day is the same old same old, you know? You get bored." This comment suggested that he enjoyed deeper relationships with the boys and counselors, and that the time he spent with them went beyond a boring daily routine.

For a few boys, an incentive program was particularly helpful. Adrian discussed the *Super-tienda* program that was enacted in the transition home, explaining that when you demonstrate certain values, like "honesty, kindness, being helpful," you can earn tokens with which you can buy things in the campus store. "I have a ton!" he said proudly, but so far he has not redeemed them, which suggests that their value may be more than their purchasing power. Tito liked the "Rally" program. "That's where you earn money if you behave and if you do all of your chores. . . . When I would do things well, they would tell me I earned more points and then I could earn money to buy myself something. It made me want to do the things I had to do." These programmatic initiatives seemed to inspire a sense of pride associated with meeting obligations and demonstrating desired attitudes and behaviors, and the rewards served as additional motivation.

Other boys talked about the "godparent" program as especially meaningful. Throughout the Esperanza Program's development, various individuals from sponsoring institutions in the United States have visited the homes in La Paz and built relationships with the some of the boys. Some have become "godparents" to some of the boys and continue to correspond with them via letters.

Since getting an education was often viewed as the key means to "become somebody," educational opportunities served as a central source of motivation. For a few boys, learning was simply enjoyable and they were excited by the new challenges they encountered in school. As Lucho explained, "I felt really good studying. When the teacher went fast, I liked going fast, too, because I felt fulfilled. I was getting ahead." Lucho was stimulated by his learning experiences in the classroom of the transition home and was excited by the possibility of enrolling in school. Not wanting to lose that possibility helped him to stay in the home and not run back to the streets. "I wanted to learn," he said, "so I didn't want to leave. . . . They were saying that if I tried hard, I would be able to go to school." Other boys saw enrolling in school as a major step in their transition process, but had some trepidation at the prospect. "I was really happy about it," said Adrian about entering public school, "but I also lost a few years. So, I'm supposed to be in eighth grade, but I'm only in fifth now." Nevertheless, he felt being enrolled in school was better than being in the remedial program in the home (primarily for the extra social opportunities) and he talked about this move as a major accomplishment. It seemed he and several other boys saw a direct connection between the years they needed to make up in school and their level of transition success. It almost was as if each year of school they could make up would erase a year lost on the streets, giving education a certain power of redemption.

Finally, the boys' accounts of what helped the transition process were notably future oriented. In this way, they stood in sharp contrast to the boys' accounts of their lives in their original homes and their lives on the streets. While arguably this could be due to the simple fact that they are now older than they were when they were with their families or on the streets, the boys clearly felt motivated by certain goals they had or promises they saw in the future. Focusing on those goals and possibilities helped them resist the temptation to run back to the streets and commit to stabilizing in the home. When Florentino and another boy were talking about running away, counselors helped them envision how their futures would be affected by whatever choice they made. Viewing the future in such a tangible way was a new experience for Florentino; one that had a profound effect on him and helped prevent his return to the streets. Damian said he realized that staying in the home "was really going to open doors for me. First, I'd have to learn to behave myself and obviously that would open doors for me. . . . But when they talked to us about going to college . . . that really excited me." During his time in the Esperanza Program, he has thought often about finishing high school and going on to college. "More than anything that's been my goal," he explained, "and it has motivated me to keep going." Diego was similarly motivated. Referring to Esperanza's plans to open a special dormitory-like facility to support boys during higher education and in their transition to independence, he said "It really excited us when they talked about the apartments. It really excited all of us to think that we would be able to continue studying."

Excitement about the future gave some of the boys a distinct determination to succeed. They were determined to accomplish primarily educational goals for the identity enhancements they would bring, but also to be able to demonstrate their capability to others. They hoped to impress their family members, but they also talked about wanting to prove something to society, as well.

A FRAMEWORK FOR TRANSITION SUCCESS

The boys identified a variety of factors—behavioral changes, spiritual transformation, academic achievement, rules and responsibilities, plans for the future, and being able to experience success and observe their own progress—that they believe contributed to their transition success. However, the set of related constructs that were indirectly, but strongly evident across discussions was their relationships in working with program staff and the climate that the institution as a whole espoused about relationships and the positive value of each human being. It was not unusual for the boys to begin their explanations of what enabled their transition success with, "My counselor told me that . . ." or "Whenever I would get frustrated, my house dad . . ." Yet, when directly asked, they credited the skill or the lesson with facilitating the process. Interestingly, though the boys did not tend to describe their relationships with adults or their peers in the residential program as central to their process of transitioning off of the streets, they did directly claim that the difference between the residential program and their original homes had much to do with relationships. The boys claimed that their family members "didn't really know them" or that they "had no control" or that they were not involved in their lives. This disconnect seems important, especially considering that family members often offered lessons and endorsed values consistent with those promoted in the residential program.

The boys spoke at length about the lessons they learned in the residential program and demonstrated a sense of ownership over the values they claimed to have learned there. The Esperanza Program consciously attempts to promote certain values (words like honesty, integrity, kindness, and respect decorate the walls of the homes with pictures illustrating their social value).

In similar ways, this is what facilitated the function of the protective supports being offered by the Esperanza Program. Though each support, whether it was educational assistance, rules and boundaries, or an incentive program, had value in its own right, they were all embedded within a relational context that seemed to enable their coordination and unleash their power. As part of their transition process, the boys developed a new identity that was embedded in a relationship with the caregivers and the program itself. Though at times they were tempted or compelled to give in to "street" values and behavior, they became increasingly unwilling to break the relationship they had developed with the program and its agents because it was intricately connected to their new identity.

In a recent study, Aronowitz (2005) attempted to identify the mechanism of resilience among youth who participated in risk-taking behaviors. The grounded theory that emerged from her research lends support to the idea that protective factors can be activated through relationships. Her findings build upon the well-established notion that relationships with caring adults can play an important role in mediating risk (Aronowitz, 2005; Rhodes, 2002). They suggest that relationships serve as the context through which risk-taking youth can envision the future and acquire the motivation to reduce their risk-taking behaviors. This happens as those relationships provide modeling, monitoring, and coaching, and as they help counter stereotypes, increasing feelings of competence and raising expectations of the youth. These specific findings are reminiscent of themes that emerged from this study. Three responses to this relational exchange seem to characterize the boys after successful transition: hope, trust, and personal agency.

First and foremost, the transition process was about hope. Admittedly, the amount of hope the boys had when they first entered the residential program was just enough to get them through the front door, but not enough to possess any degree of expectation. Over time, however, increased hope developed as boys were helped to examine future possibilities. As they observed and experienced opportunities for positive self-development (opportunities like educational support or interaction with foreign visitors, for example) they became more committed to their own futures and were hopeful about their prospects for success. Thus hope both facilitated and was facilitated by greater future orientation and knowledge of specific resources and opportunities. Increased hope then fed into the larger system of faith and relationship. As hope increased, faith in the transition process was bolstered and boys were more willing to trust in their relationship to the program and its agents. Hope was further supported by religious values, specifically the belief that faith would bring reward. Several boys expressed this belief in the literal sense, referring to the Christian concept of justification, or the idea that salvation would be granted to those who have faith. Most, however, focused more generally on the idea that God would reward ongoing efforts of self-improvement; if they worked hard, they could earn a diploma, get a good job, and be able to provide for their families.

Trust was another key part of the transition process. In order to experience success, the boys' faith in what might be possible required them to trust in others, trust in the programmatic system, and trust in themselves. As they experienced their caregivers and the programmatic promises as trustworthy, they experienced themselves as worthy of respect and investment. Over time, these relational experiences of trust fueled increased faith in the transition process and strengthened the relational context that supported and contained the boys' new identities as children who had left the streets. Lucho shared a powerful comment about the function and value of trust when he said that trusting helped him develop deeper relationships, and as he did he felt "like I had my own home."

It is tempting to think that the family environment offered to the boys through the Esperanza Program became real for them over time and that their adopted new home was a preferable replacement for the original. If the boys had not spoken so often about their strong desires for connection to their original families, we might have been more willing to believe this idea. What Lucho means here, and what the boys in general feel, is that through the process of transitioning, they became part of a relational system that helped them develop a new and stable identity. This new identity was characterized by certain values, beliefs, and experiences associated with healthy life off the streets and was supported by the shared caring and moral belief between the boys and their caregivers. Lucho, the other boys, and their caregivers all believed in the promise and value of transitioning off of the streets and they all had faith that success was possible. Lucho felt like he had his own home because he had a deeper sense of who he was and who he wanted to be, and that was rooted in a consistent and consuming system. There was synchrony between what Lucho believed he could do and be and what those around him believed. When family members entered into this system and reestablished relationships with the boys, they became a part of this synchrony and their presence lent exponential power to the boys' commitment and ultimate success.

A final component of the transition process had to do with personal agency. A subset of the protective factors and experiences recalled by the boys related to skills and abilities they developed. As they acquired more adaptive social skills, as they learned how to follow a schedule and were reintegrated into school, and as they learned concrete lessons that helped them better understand the value of things like respect and hard work, they developed an increasing sense of personal agency. They began to see how they could act as agents in their own world and control certain elements of their own existence. For example, boys often spoke about understanding that if they studied hard and applied themselves at school, they would be able to graduate and obtain employment. They also began to understand concepts like "respect breeds respect," and the results they saw when they applied this wisdom reinforced the idea that they could potentially influence how others might respond to them. Experiences like these helped them develop an internal locus of control, which has frequently been associated with increased resilience across populations at risk (Luthar & Zigler, 1991; Rutter, 1987).

DISCUSSION

Findings related to the backgrounds of the boys and the experiences they had prior to moving to the streets confirm the findings of prior research and add important new details. Poverty, maltreatment, and domestic violence have proven to be common factors in the families of children who end up living on the streets (Bond, 1993; Scanlon et al., 1998) and they were common factors in the backgrounds of the participants of this study, as well. Likewise, movement onto the streets was the result of a combination of previously documented "push" and "pull" factors.

The reasons boys gave for being in the streets—primarily the abuse and neglect in their homes and the opportunities for diversion, socialization and economic opportunity on the streets—are relevant to understanding their trajectories but alone provide only a limited picture of what occurred. As the boys shared their experiences, a central story emerged that, while not true in every way for every participant, communicates complex and multilayered struggles that implicate the need for various levels of intervention. Findings demonstrated that, although the boys' families contributed to their existence on the streets in the first place, they also played a significant role in helping the boys transition off of the streets. In some cases, the families served as motivation for their transition success. Some of the boys wanted to succeed so they could help their families in the future, while others wanted to make them proud of their accomplishments. In other cases, families provided more direct support, visiting boys in the program and encouraging their progress. Thus a key finding of this study was that families played an important role in the boys' transitions both onto *and* off of the streets. This finding echoes findings in the research on runaway and homeless youth in North America, which identified family members as key helping resources in youths' transitions off of the streets (Kurtz et al., 2000; Lindsey et al., 2000).

Noticeably absent from the literature on street children is the role of schools. We know from the considerable body of research on resilience that activities and supports outside of the home can serve as powerful buffers to the risks associated with family dysfunction and poverty (Luthar & Zigler, 1991; Rutter, 1987; Scales & Leffert, 1999). Schools, as mandated participants in the lives of children, have an unparalleled opportunity to provide a buffering effect and are therefore frequently a focus in the discussion on how to promote youth resilience (Scales & Leffert, 1999). Yet, their role has rarely, if ever, been examined in the experiences of street children. This study revealed that school and educational achievement are significant factors in the transitions of children onto and off of the streets. All but one of the boys in this study had neutral or negative experiences in school prior to leaving home and frequently opted to skip classes to pursue other activities on the streets. For them, school was not a positive alternative to their homes and it frequently contributed additional stresses like bullies, academic failure, and punishment for misbehavior. The one boy who did have a positive school experience prior to running to the streets had a strikingly different overall trajectory from the others, which suggests that school may have played an influential role.

Despite the negative feelings about school the rest of the boys had before and during their time on the streets, all possessed a firm belief that education was a way to "become somebody." Experiencing success in the classroom or reaching important milestones like being reintegrated into school helped boost their self-esteem and reinforce the notion that they were no longer "nothings." In difficult moments when the temptation to run back to the streets was great, it was often the thought of losing educational opportunities or standing that convinced them to stay. They found strength in the promises offered by educational achievement: they could become someone, they could make their parents proud, and as employed professionals, they could have the financial means to help their families. As a powerful variable, educational achievement thus has the potential either to bolster a boy's transition success, or threaten it, if he experiences failure in his educational pursuits during the transition process.

Another difference between the findings of the runaway youth literature and the findings of this study involves helping resources. In the former, helping resources are frequently discussed as primarily human resources (Bender et al., 2007; Kidd & Davidson, 2007; Kurtz et al., 2000; Lindsey et al., 2000). Former runaways tend to focus less on program details and more on the quality of relationships they have with helpers when discussing what enabled their successful transitions. Though human support was a category that emerged in the boys' stories of what they found helpful in the transition process, programmatic support emerged as a theme of equal importance. Many boys viewed the structured schedule, boundaries and rules, and daily responsibilities of the transition program as especially helpful. Some also mentioned incentive programs, through which they could earn rewards for either demonstrating positive behaviors or completing chores. These programmatic elements seem to have contributed a sense of stability, upon which boys could measure their progress and achieve a degree of control. Their increasing ability to master the challenges set out in the transition program—challenges like completing homework and chores, and respecting others and not fighting—helped them feel more grounded in their lives off of the streets and oriented them toward the possibilities of the future.

The ability to focus on the future was strongly associated with transition success in the boys' stories of their experiences. The more boys developed a future orientation and began to imagine concrete aspects of how their lives might unfold, the more they were motivated to commit to the transition process. As they moved forward achieving goals that were set for them by the program, or that they set for themselves, they felt less connected to their lives on the streets and even more focused on continued achievement. It was only after the boys began experiencing some success off the streets that they seemed to develop the strong determination discussed in the runaway youth literature as a critical personal attribute in resilience.

IMPLICATIONS FOR RESEARCH AND PRACTICE

The results of this work bear some important implications for both research and practice. Since the body of literature on street children is still so limited, there are many opportunities for further research. In general, research needs to expand beyond defining the problems of street children from various angles and begin exploring pathways toward different solutions. Additional qualitative research is needed to build upon the findings of this study and explore the experiences of other groups of children who have successfully transitioned off of the streets. Comparative studies of children with similar backgrounds who do and do not leave home would help us identify more discrete sources of risk and resilience, as would comparative studies of children who do and do not choose to leave the streets. Finally, given the very limited successes that practitioners see relative to the numbers of lost children, practice-based research would provide an opportunity to examine more closely the strategies currently being used to intervene in the lives of street children and identify potential areas for improvement or change.

This work bears implications for practice on multiple levels. First, findings from this study reveal opportunities for preventive practice. Certainly, intervention efforts directed at families to help stem intrafamilial violence and teach more effective and humane disciplinary strategies might make a substantial difference in preventing the flow of children onto the streets. Additionally, programs that engage children and provide stimulating activities and social opportunities during out-of-school time could make a substantial difference by occupying many of the hours children are currently spending looking for stimulation and socialization on the streets. Another opportunity highlighted by this study involves the school as a potential source of support. There is promise in the idea that schools could participate in identifying children at increased risk of being on the streets and collaborate with other service providers to offer preventive supports of various forms.

For practitioners providing intervention services for those already living on the streets, this study offers some particular suggestions. Transitioning off of the streets seems to require intensive and constant relational and structural supports. Having counselors and other staff members available at all hours to provide real-time support to children in crisis moments may limit returns to the streets and contribute to the development of important transition-related skills. Opportunities to see the future in concrete ways, experience achievement, and measure progress can help reinforce the transition process in ways that promote greater commitment and determination. Given the substantial value boys seemed to place on educational achievement, the provision of supports to enable success in this area would likely accomplish far more than just academic progress.

The significance of family cannot be underestimated. Practitioners should explore how family members could be involved to help support the transition process. Though it is likely many children will continue to need residential care into adulthood, opportunities for family reintegration, possibly involving shared responsibilities for care with support programs, should be examined.

Finally, it is recommended that practitioners attend to the relational and spiritual lives of the children in their care, since both of these factors play a powerful role in helping children transform their lives. More research is needed to explore exactly how this might be done in the most respectful and healthy ways. However, at a minimum, rituals or activities designed to help promote forgiveness, activate deeper consciousness, encourage moral development, and foster more future-oriented thinking might prove beneficial.

As Ungar et al. (2007) stated, "Resilience is not a permanent state of being, but a condition of becoming better" (p. 301). The boys stepped into relationship with the Esperanza Program and their counselors when they entered the transition home. They took a leap of faith that this decision would be fruitful. Their faith involved elements of hope (that this move would bring some benefit), and trust (that the people would deliver on their promises and that what they offered would be valid and worthwhile), and it was strengthened and deepened as the boys developed a sense of personal agency that in turn supported their ongoing faith development. There were blips in this process to be sure. In those moments when the boys were ready to run back to the streets, when their faith in the transition process waned, their relationships to their caregivers came into direct play. The caregivers reminded the boys of their connection to the transition process. As they tried to dissuade the boys from giving up, they evoked hopeful images of the future, they pointed out ways in which their trust in the system had been honored, and they asked the boys to make their own decisions after thoughtful reflection.

REFERENCES

Anarfi, J. (1997). Vulnerability to sexually transmitted disease: Street children in Accra. *Health Transition Review, 7*(Suppl.), 281–306.

Aronowitz, T. (2005). The role of "envisioning the future" in the development of resilience among at-risk youth. *Public Health Nursing, 22*(3), 200–208.

Bender, K., Thompson, S., McManus, H., Lantry, J., & Flynn, P. (2007). Capacity for survival: Strengths of homeless street youth. *Child Youth Care Forum, 36*, 25–42.

Bond, L. (1993). La dolorosa realidad de los niños de la calle. *Boletin de la Oficina Sanitaria Panamericana, 114*(2), 97–101.

Diversi, M., Moraes Filho, N., & Morelli, M. (1999). Daily reality on the streets of Campinas, Brazil. In M. Raffaelli and R. W. Larson (Eds.), *Homeless and working youth around the world: Exploring developmental issues* (pp. 19–34). San Francisco: Jossey-Bass.

Domic, J., & Ardaya, G. (1991). *Los menores de Bolivia sujetos sociales hoy o mañana: Analisis de situación de niños en circunstancias especialmente difíciles*. La Paz, Bolivia: Fundación San Gabriel.

Dybicz, P. (2005). Interventions for street children: An analysis of current best practices. *International Social Work, 48*(6), 763–771.

Earls, F., & Carlson, M. (1999). Children at the margins of society: Research and practice. In M. Raffaelli & R. W. Larson (Eds.), *Homeless and working children around the world: Exploring developmental issues* (pp. 71–82). San Francisco: Jossey-Bass.

Ferguson, C., McIntyre, L., & Kaminsky, D. (1993). Opiniones de los adultos Hondureños respecto a los niños callejeros. *Boletin de la Oficina Sanitaria Panamericana, 114*(2), 105–114.

Hecht, T. (1998). *At home in the street: Street children of northeast Brazil*. Cambridge: Cambridge University Press.

Huang, C. (1998). Characterization of the health and social environment of the street children of La Paz, Bolivia (Unpublished medical school thesis). Harvard Medical School, Cambridge, MA.

Hutz, C. S., & Koller, S. H. (1999). Methodological and ethical issues in research with street children. *New Directions for Child and Adolescent Development, 85*, 59–70.

Inciardi, J., & Surratt, H. (1998). Children in the streets of Brazil: Drug use, crime, violence and HIV risks. *Substance Use & Misuse, 33*(7), 1461–1480.

Kidd, S., & Davidson, L. (2007). "You have to adapt because you have no other choice": The stories of strength and resilience of 208 homeless youth in New York City and Toronto. *Journal of Community Psychology, 35*(2), 219–238.

Kleiber, P. (2004). Focus groups: More than a method of qualitative inquiry. In K. DeMarrais & S. Lapan (Eds.), *Foundations for research: Methods of inquiry in education and the social sciences* (pp. 87–102). Mahwah, NJ: Lawrence Erlbaum Associates.

Kurtz, P., Lindsey, E., Jarvis, S., & Nackerud, L. (2000). How runaway and homeless youth navigate the troubled waters: The role of formal and informal helpers. *Child & Adolescent Social Work Journal, 17*(5), 381–402.

Lalor, K. (1999). Street children: A comparative perspective. *Child Abuse & Neglect, 23*(8), 759–770.

Lindsey, E., Kurtz, P. D., Jarvis, S., Williams, N., & Nackerud, L. (2000). How runaway and homeless youth navigate troubled waters: Personal strengths and resources. *Child & Adolescent Social Work Journal, 17*(2), 115–140.

Luthar, S., & Zigler, E. (1991). Vulnerability and competence: A review of research on resilience in childhood. *American Journal of Orthopsychiatry, 61,* 6–22.

MacKnee, C., & Mervyn, J. (2002). Critical incidents that facilitate homeless people's transition off the streets. *Journal of Social Distress and the Homeless, 11*(4), 293–306.

Miles, M. B., & Huberman, A. M. (1994). *Qualitative data analysis* (2nd ed.). Thousand Oaks, CA: Sage.

Molnar, B., Shade, S., Kral, A., Booth, R., & Watters, J. (1998). Suicidal behavior and sexual/physical abuse among street youth. *Child Abuse & Neglect, 22*(3), 213–222.

Rew, L., Taylor-Seehafer, M., Thomas, N., & Yockey, R. (2001). Correlates of resilience in homeless adolescents. *Journal of Nursing Scholarship, 33*(1), 33–40.

Rhodes, J. (2002). *Stand by me: The risks and rewards of mentoring today's youth.* Cambridge, MA: Harvard University Press.

Rutter, M. (1987). Psychosocial resilience and protective mechanisms. *American Journal of Orthopsychiatry, 57,* 316–331.

Scales, P., & Leffert, N. (1999). *Developmental assets: A synthesis of the scientific research on adolescent development.* Minneapolis, MN: Search Institute.

Scanlon, T., Tomkins, A., Lynch, M., & Scanlon, F. (1998). Street children in Latin America. *British Medical Journal, 316,* 1596–1600.

Strauss, A., & Corbin, A. (1998). *Basics of qualitative research.* Thousand Oaks, CA: Sage.

Ungar, M., Brown, M., Liebenberg, L., Othman, R., Kwong, W., Armstrong, M., et al. (2007). Unique pathways to resilience across cultures. *Adolescence, 42*(166), 287–310.

UNICEF-Bolivia. (1994). *La niñez y la mujer en Bolivia: Analisis de situación.* La Paz, Bolivia: UNICEF.

United Nations. (1986). *The situation of youth in the 1980's and prospects and challenges for the year 2000.* New York: Department of International Economics and Social Affairs, United Nations.

Vaughn, S., Schumm, J. S., & Sinagub, J. M. (1996). *Focus group interviews in education and psychology.* Thousand Oaks, CA: Sage.

Veeran, V. (2004). Working with street children: A child centered approach. *Child Care in Practice, 10*(4), 359–366.

Williams, C. (1993). Who are "street children"? A hierarchy of street use and appropriate responses. *Child Abuse & Neglect, 17*, 831–841.

Williams, N., Lindsey, E., Kurtz, P., & Jarvis, S. (2001). From trauma to resiliency: Lessons from former runaway and homeless youth. *Journal of Youth Studies, 4*(2), 233–253.

Wittig, M., Wright, J., & Kaminsky, D. (1997). Substance abuse among street children in Honduras. *Substance Use & Misuse, 32*(7–8), 805–827.

Wright, J., Kaminsky, D., & Wittig, M. (1993). Health and social conditions of street children in Honduras. *American Journal of Disadvantaged Children, 147*, 279–283.

Chapter 2

CHALLENGES AND OPPORTUNITIES: IMPROVING EARLY CHILDHOOD DEVELOPMENT IN SOUTH AFRICA

Andrew Dawes and Linda Biersteker

It is well established that the early years are a particularly sensitive period. Brain and biological development in the early years is experienced based, leading to neurophysiological pathways being laid down in synaptic formations in the brain (Young & Mustard, 2008). These establish the foundation for emotional, language, motor and cognitive competencies. The quality of sensitivity provided in early relationships with caregivers is integral to this process. The developmental sensitivity of this period provides both opportunities for laying a positive foundation for the child's future emotional and intellectual development, as well as being a time during which developmental insults can have a long lasting impact. Interventions to support a sound early start and limit vulnerability is particularly important in resource compromised communities such as prevail in South Africa (Engel et al., 2007; Richter, 2004).

South Africa presents a particularly interesting case study of a middle income developing country that is attempting to grapple with the challenge of improving early childhood outcomes in the context of a society in transition, a relatively low skill base, long-term structural inequality, high levels of interpersonal violence, and the ravages of the HIV pandemic (Republic of South Africa, 2009).

It is perhaps not sufficiently appreciated that the after the country's liberation in 1994 (a mere 16 years ago), a legal and policy revolution had to be undertaken. The new state inherited racist legislation and policy that applied to children—all had to change. Racially divided health, education, and social welfare systems and their bureaucracies had to be integrated. Five additional provincial governments were established with responsibilities for implementing national policy in matters affecting children (e.g., health, education, and welfare). These were huge undertakings and they are still being completed; for example, the Children's Act (No. 38 of 2005 as Amended 2007) legislation that seeks to promote children's welfare and development. South Africa's first guidelines for Child and Adolescent Mental Health were published in 2003, and the post Apartheid Mental Health Act (which has minimal reference to children) was promulgated in 2006 (Flisher et al., in press).

The Children's Act is the most important piece of legislation in regard to provision for early childhood and child protection. It recognizes the importance of early intervention and the vulnerability of young children. Its central objectives are to "promote the protection, development and well-being of children." The Act also makes extensive provision for early childhood development services and for child protection interventions.

The Act is a wide ranging piece of legislation, and a major advance on the earlier law. It is anchored firmly in a child rights framework, and establishes the responsibilities of government and those who care for children, particularly the most vulnerable. However, regulations, standards and procedures remain to be finalized rendering the implementation of policy an uncertain process.

The most important policy document in recent years is the National Integrated Plan for Early Childhood Development (NIP for ECD) (Departments of Education, Health, and Social Development, 2005). The NIP recognizes key threats to early health and psychological development and outlines a range of commitments to improving services to children under five years of age (Biersteker & Kvalsvig, 2007). The NIP specifically targets the poorest and most vulnerable children for intervention, recognizing that it is this sector of the child population that requires the most support. The NIP emphasizes a holistic approach to improving child well-being, strengthening human capital outcomes, and reducing threats to healthy development.

The NIP for ECD policy states (Departments of Education, Health, and Social Development, 2005, p. 17):

Ultimately, the integrated intersectoral ECD should

- create environments and situations in which children, particularly vulnerable children, can learn, grow and thrive socially, emotionally, physically and cognitively;
- increase the opportunities for young children to prepare for entering formal schooling;

- provide support to adults who care for young children and the communities in which they live, in order to enhance their abilities to care for and educate these children; and
- reduce the adverse developmental effects of poverty and other forms of deprivation on children from zero to four.

This is an ambitious policy initiative. Its primary locus of delivery is in local sites, be they clinics, ECD centers and the range of home-based interventions currently offered with the NGO sector. There are many challenges in delivering on this promise. We point to some ways in which evidence and appropriate evaluation can strengthen delivery and impact on child mental health.

South Africa's burst of child policy making energy had its roots in a strong civil society movement that fought for child rights and protection during resistance to apartheid. That history as challenging as it was, provided a significant opportunity to place children at the fore of the policy making process. The continuing challenge is to realize the goals of fine law and policy in the face of multiple threats to the well-being of young children.

The remainder of this chapter proceeds from a brief outline of the contexts of children's development in the country, to a consideration of the major threats to well-being in a developing country such as South Africa and finally to a discussion of four promising initiatives that seek to address them. The focus will be on prevention of adverse experience and promotion of sound development.

EARLY CHILD DEVELOPMENT IN SOUTH AFRICA

ECD is defined as in South Africa as

an umbrella term that applies to the processes by which children from birth to about nine years grow and thrive, physically, mentally, emotionally, spiritually, morally and socially. (Department of Education, 2001, p. 3)

While the period extends to nine years, the chapter will focus on the under fives. Major contextual influences on the quality the early childhood environment for the majority of South African children are described in this section. They include population structure, income distribution and poverty, the major causes of morbidity and mortality for adults and children, and the educational environment for young children. The reader who wishes to have more detailed information on household and child statistics is referred to http://www.statssa.gov.za/ or http://childrencount.ci.org.za/ and to the Development Indicators report of the South African Presidency (Republic of South Africa, 2009).

POPULATION

It is inappropriate to speak of a single South African childhood. These are many and varied: significant, though unknown numbers of children grow up on the streets; others live in rural subsistence agriculture communities that uphold traditional African ways of life, while the majority live in cities and towns (see later). South Africa has eleven official Languages and at least twice as many are spoken in the smaller ethnolinguistic communities (including migrants and refugees from the north). Children grow up in a number of religious communities, the largest being Christian, but with significant minorities of the Muslim, Hindu, and Jewish faiths (Statistics South Africa, 1999). In 2009 the South African population[1] was estimated to be 49.32 million (Statistics South Africa, 2009a).

Many children growing up in towns and cities retain strong connections with their rural roots as children of recently urbanized families may shuttle between town and country at different points in their lives. Statistics on the matter are not available, but in the authors' experience, it is common for a mother in town to send her child to the countryside for primary school, and for the child to return to the town for senior schooling due to limited facilities in the countryside, or in anticipation that she will receive a better education.

The child population disaggregated by "race"[2] is displayed in Table 2.1. It is important to disaggregate early childhood to those over and under five years of age as the latter is a particularly sensitive time in the life cycle. Just as there are huge opportunities during this developmental period for laying sound platforms for children's future development, insults to health and development can also have long lasting impacts (Engel et al., 2007; Grantham-McGregor et al., 2007).

Table 2.1
South African child population

	Child population under 18 years N (% of total South African population)	Child population under 9 years N (% of total South African population)	Child population under 5 years N (% of total South African population)
Black	19,594,400	9,742,800	4,820,200
White	1,120,600	510,700	248,700

INCOME DISTRIBUTION AND POVERTY

Poverty presents a range of risks to early childhood development, particularly in the earliest years (Aber & Bennett, 1997). Due to a range of factors, including the policies of the white minority government prior to 1994, a poorly educated young population, high unemployment, and limited economic growth, the vast majority of children live in poverty (the white minority is minimally affected) (Republic of South Africa, 2009). South Africa does not have consensus on the measurement of poverty. A commonly accepted poverty line is those living in the poorest 40% of all households. Based on this metric, and using the 2005 Income and Expenditure Survey, Streak, Yu, and van der Berg (2008) estimate that 65% of all children (11.8 million) live in poverty, with 66% of those aged zero to four having this status. Clearly a vast number are vulnerable to the broad impact of poverty.

There is no state unemployment benefit in South Africa. However, the government is committed to assisting as far as possible. Parents with children under 15 years of age who have an income of less than about US$307 per month can claim a Child Support Grant valued at US$30 per month (December 2009 values). Current estimates suggest that 82% of South African children are eligible (Budlender, 2008).

Notwithstanding social grant income, South Africa is currently the most unequal society in the world with a Gini coefficient[3] estimated at between 0.66 and 0.68 depending on the survey (Republic of South Africa, 2009). The Human Development Index (HDI) in 2007–2008 was 0.674 ranking South Africa 121 of 177 nations.

MORBIDITY AND MORTALITY

Despite free treatment available to children under six years of age and high levels of immunization, those zero to four years are especially vulnerable to illness and death and the highest number of all deaths in the population in 2005 was for this age group The official estimated infant mortality rate in 2009 is 45.7, and the Actuarial Society of South Africa model estimates the under five mortality rate to be 68 per 1,000 (Republic of South Africa, 2009). Infant mortality data is not reliable as only 82% of birth registrations are current (Statistics South Africa, 2007).

AIDS related illness is the leading cause of all child deaths (40%), with diarrhea, lower respiratory infections and low birth weight accounting for a further 27% (Bradshaw, Bourne, and Nannan, 2003). In those infected children who survive, it is likely that their neurodevelopmental status will be compromised, particularly when undernourished (Potterton and Bailieu, 2008; Sher, 2005). The estimated overall HIV prevalence rate is approximately 10.6% and the total number of people living with HIV is estimated at approximately 5.21 million. For adults aged 15–49 years who are most likely to be caring for young children, an estimated 16.7% is HIV positive (Republic of South Africa, 2009). An estimated 3.3% (300,000) of children aged 2–14 years is HIV positive (Shisana et al., 2005). As it uses a method to detect *recent* infection (and therefore not transmission from mother to child), the finding indicates that children older than two years are likely to have been infected through other pathways including sexual assault (Relhe et al., 2007).

Adult mortality contributes significantly to orphaning. Current estimates by the Actuarial Society of South Africa indicate that 1.5 million South African children are orphans as a consequence of parental death due to AIDS related illnesses (http://www.healthlink.org.za/healthstats/89/data/).

Two of the most significant threats to the well-being of young children posed by the AIDS pandemic are caregiver illness and death (Brandt, Dawes, & Bray, 2006). The illness of the caregiver commonly results in an inability to work, with the associated economic shock contributing to impoverishment. As important is that ill carers are not able to provide sensitive care and stimulation to young children (Richter, 2004).

Apart from the distress caused by the death of primary caregivers, the care arrangements are bound to change, with fostering by kin or others being common outcomes when there is nobody else in the household who can look after the child. A variant of this situation occurs when there are no adults in the household and the young child is cared for by older siblings, likely to be a suboptimal arrangement for both parties and likely to compromise the developmental opportunities of both. It is not uncommon for these young caregivers to have had to look after their sick parents prior to their death (Cluver & Gardiner, 2007; Cluver, Gardiner, & Operario, 2007). Interventions to prevent the spread of HIV are clearly crucial not only to reduce the numbers of those infected, but also to reduce the risks of emotional distress and psychological disorder that may arise from parental mortality or having to live with and care for a sick parent (see later).

Vaccinations are a crucial in preventing serious medical conditions in childhood. In 2008, 88% of children were fully immunized in the first year of life, 2% short of the target for the year (Republic of South Africa, 2009).

HUNGER AND NUTRITION

Nutritional status impacts significantly on child health and well-being. It is a serious concern in South Africa, where the most recent national survey indicates that 18% of children under nine years are stunted and almost 10% are underweight. Children under four are most affected with 23% stunted and 11% underweight (Kruger, Swart, Labadarios, Dannhauser, & Nel, 2007). Close to 9% (8.9%) of children have low birth weight status, which is associated with compromised nutritional status later on. These are national aggregated figures. In areas of deep long-term poverty, much higher rates are likely to be evident. Undernutrition is an even more serious problem in children with HIV infection, where more than half become stunted or underweight and one in five develops wasting (Hendricks, Eley, & Bourne, 2006).

Stunting is associated with developmental delay and is the strongest predictor of childhood mortality in children under the age of five (ACC/SCN, 1997; Pelletier, 1994). The condition has negative consequences for human capital development as early stunting and undernutrition compromise neurological development and hinder the ability of the child to benefit from education (Walker et al., 2007).

The wastage of human capacity occasioned by this easily preventable condition is significant. This is a key area for preventive intervention in early childhood and will be addressed later in the chapter.

DISABILITY AND PSYCHIATRIC DISORDERS

Accurate figures on the proportion of children with disabilities are not available. The estimated moderate to severe disability prevalence rate for all children is between 3.3% and 8.4%, depending on the measure, and for those under 5 it is 3% (Schneider & Saloojee, 2007). Incidence in rural areas may be as high as 8.3% in children under 10 years of age (Couper, 2002).

No representative prevalence surveys of child psychiatric disorders have been conducted. Based on research in other countries and on expert opinion, it is estimated that between 15% and 17% of South Africans under 18 years are likely to suffer from a psychiatric disorder at some point (intellectual disability accounts for 2% to 3% of the total) (Kleintjies et al., 2006). There are no estimates for children under age nine. The vast majority of affected children are unlikely to be able to access a mental health service as these are few and far between.

THE RISK OF MALTREATMENT

South African society is very tolerant of violence in the domestic sphere (Jewkes, Levin, & Penn-Kekana, 2002). Internationally, young children under five years of age are particularly at risk for maltreatment (Finkelhor, 2008; Cawson, Wattam, Brooker, & Kelly, 2000), and South African studies suggest a similar trend. Prevalence and incidence estimates for children under five years are not available in South Africa (Dawes & Mushwana, 2007). However, a series of studies conducted at the Red Cross Children's Hospital in Cape Town over a period of years provides some indication in the case of young children referred for traumatic injury: 66% of children referred for serious nonaccidental injuries had been sexually assaulted. In the case of physical maltreatment 56% of cases were in children under five years; the median age of assaulted children was two years; 66% of children treated for nonaccidental injury had been sexually assaulted (Dawes & Ward, 2008; Fieggen et al., 2004; Naidoo, 2000).

Police records notoriously underestimate maltreatment, but can provide some indication of the problem (Richter & Dawes, 2008). Nationally, children constitute half the victims of reported rape and indecent assault, and 10% of assaults are perpetrated on children; the specialist police unit that deals with child maltreatment opened more than 40,000 dockets in 2004. Figures for young children are not available.

Partner violence is another serious threat to the well-being of young children. It is well known that their emotional development is compromised by exposure to violence between their caregivers (World Health Organization & ISPCAN, 2006). Representative prevalence studies indicate that at least 20% of adults are involved in violent relationships, placing significant numbers of South African children at risk for psychological problems (Dawes, de Sas Kropiwnicki, Kafaar, & Richter, 2006; Jewkes et al., 2002).

EARLY EDUCATION

The poverty environments within which most South African children grow up do not provide good platforms for cognitive development and full participation in society. Nowhere is this more evident than in this country's poor schooling outcomes and low skills base. Against this background increasing access to early childhood education opportunities has become a policy priority in South Africa. This includes phasing in of a reception year of schooling (grade R) for all five-year-olds as well as a commitment to increasing access to educational stimulation through a variety of programs for younger children (Department of Education, 2001; Departments of Education, Health, and Social Development, 2005). Schooling is compulsory in the year children turn seven.

Accurate information on enrollment in ECD programs is not available for children under school going age. Estimates based on the General

Household Survey 2008 (Statistics South Africa, 2009b) suggest that 17% of children under five years access an ECD program.

Fifty-two percent of children attended grade R classes in primary schools in 2008 and 68% of grade 1 learners had attended preschool programs the previous year suggesting that another 16% of learners attended community-based grade R classes (personal communication, Monitoring and Evaluation Directorate, National Department of Education, 2009). Ninety-four percent of children (six to nine years) are enrolled in grades 1–3 at primary schools (personal communication, Monitoring and Evaluation Directorate, National Department of Education, 2009).

Though access to early education is increasing, the quality of services is variable and the capacity of many children to benefit is undermined by undernutrition, poor health and inadequate caregiving.

National assessments of literacy and numeracy are cause for concern with mean scores in grade 3 of 36% and 35% for literacy and numeracy, respectively (Department of Education, 2008). Improving the quality of education particularly in the early stages is a major concern for the Department and a number of initiatives have been put in place to address this (Biersteker, 2009).

We have described a range of risks to the well-being of a significant proportion of young South African children. The manner in which they operate to influence developmental outcomes is illustrated in Figure 2.1. We have added *caregiver health and well-being*, a mediating variable which is of critical importance in all development, but particularly in South Africa as a consequence of high prevalence of HIV and AIDS and infectious diseases such as Tuberculosis (Brandt, 2007; Brandt et al., 2006; Bray & Brandt, 2007; Richter, Manegold, & Pather, 2004).

Impoverished household conditions such as those that prevail in South Africa have been shown to impact on caregiver mental status. Also, recent studies of impoverished women with depressive symptoms are demonstrating how maternal mental state impacts on infant development. For example, a study conducted in rural Bangladesh found that depressed mothers were less sensitive to their infants than controls in the same community, and that low sensitivity and maternal depressive symptoms were negatively associated with infant development (Black et al., 2007). Similar findings are emerging from South African research where one recent study indicates that *maternal depression* may be a significant problem among young mothers living in poverty in this country (Cooper et al., 2009; Tomlinson, Cooper, Stein, Swartz, & Molteno, 2006). While more research is needed in South Africa, there is no doubt that when caregiver well-being is compromised, the capacity to care for young children suffers, and child

Figure 2.1
A conceptual model of how risk factors affect early childhood psychological development

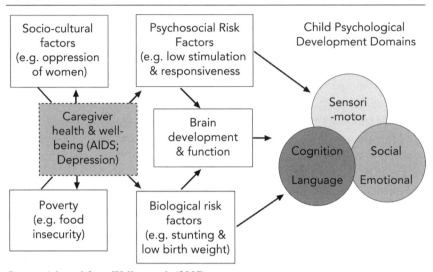

Source: Adapted from Walker et al. (2007).

outcomes including health, nutritional status, and psychological development are compromised (Richter, 2004; Richter & Grieve, 1991; Richter, 1994; Martorell, 1996).

Interventions designed to reduce risks and promote early development need to appreciate each element of this complex chain of relationships.

INTERVENTIONS

A key goal of South African ECD services is to promote good child and caregiver outcomes, and the National Integrated Plan is particularly directed to improve the situation and outcomes of children affected by poverty and related risks (Departments of Education, Health, and Social Development, 2005). There is broad agreement in South African and other sub-Saharan African countries that certain key domains should be attended to in efforts to improve early development outcomes in the face of the considerable risks to child well-being (Engel et al., 2007; Walker et al., 2007). They include the following:

1. survival
2. health (including mental health nutritional status, HIV status, developmental disability and injury)
3. psychosocial development, including motor, emotional, cognitive, and language development and social development and participation

The domains comprising the third set are all relevant to capacitation for schooling and beyond. Each component is important for current well-being as well as for building the platform for schooling. For example, the cognitive domain includes mathematical and logical thought, representation and a range of memory capacities. The language domain includes language expression, emergent literacy and several others. Children's social characteristics, the quality of their relationships with others, the extent to which they are prosocial or antisocial in orientation, the degree to which they display empathy to the vulnerable, are all a product of their early relationships with caregivers, and the quality of socialization from the family through the school. Social participation refers to their engagement in group activities such as sports or the arts, and later in life to civic and political participation.

There is a wealth of literature on all these topics. We can only touch on some aspects here. In what follows, we focus on three issues that are major challenges for children in South Africa and the rest of the sub-Saharan region (Garcia, Pence, & Evans, 2008):

1. malnutrition rehabilitation
2. addressing the impact of HIV and AIDS on the young child in low resource settings
3. child maltreatment prevention in the home
4. programming for early childhood development in the years before school

Throughout, the discussion will principally consider the preschool years.

REHABILITATION OF MALNOURISHED CHILDREN

Malnutrition is one of four major risk factors for child development identified in the 2007 Lancet Series on child development in developing countries (Grantham-McGregor et al., 2007). Given the extent of chronic malnutrition in South Africa, as described earlier, and the impact of HIV on young children's nutritional status, government has put in place an Integrated Nutrition Program (INP) which has three main components, including the following:

• health facility–based nutrition program and strategies
• community-based nutrition programs and strategies
• nutrition and HIV and AIDS support programs and strategies

These span a range of promotive, preventive, therapeutic and rehabilitative activities. At risk, pregnant and lactating women and children under five years are priority targets for the INP. Key areas include nutrition education, promotion of exclusive breast-feeding, growth monitoring, food fortification, and micronutrient supplementation as preventive strategies.

In a recent review of nutritional strategies, Swart, Sanders, and McLachlan (2008) conclude that inadequate implementation rather than inappropriate policies and strategies is the basis for limited success of these policies. The review also recommends that interventions are scaled once they have been proven to work and with sufficient accompanying resources. We provide examples of two initiatives for malnutrition rehabilitation that have been shown to be effective.

The first initiative targeted management of severe malnutrition in two rural hospitals that both had high case fatality rates for severely malnourished children (46% and 25%, respectively). It involved forming a hospital nutrition team to assess the clinical management of severe malnutrition, action plans to improve the quality of care and monitoring and evaluation of activities. These actions reduced fatality to 21% and 18%, respectively, indicating that staff motivation and training even in remote facilities can improve clinical management and the quality of care for malnourished children (Swart et al., 2008).

A study of the Philani Nutrition program in Greater Cape Town (Le Roux, 2006) shows that home-based programs can be effective in reducing malnutrition. Children below the third percentile were identified through door-to-door home visits by outreach workers who had had a three week training in nutrition, general health, growth monitoring. They had been selected following a positive deviant approach in that visitors were from the same communities and living circumstances but their children were not malnourished. Children in the program receive a medical examination, micronutrients, and deworming, and advice on breast-feeding or nutritious and locally available low cost food was provided to the mother. Outreach workers conducted follow-up visits to the household in order to monitor the mother and child/children's progress. These visits were also used to educate the mother in practical parenting skills. Le Roux's study confirmed that child care practices are a key predictor of speed of rehabilitation. The intervention succeeded in raising the weight of 53.6% of the 500 nutritionally compromised children above the third percentile within 188 days.

As has been demonstrated in other similar settings (Walker, Chang, Powell, & Grantham-McGregor, 2005; Lewin et al., 2005), this initiative indicates that with support, community level workers with relatively little formal education can work with the child's carer in the home setting to facilitate improvements in children's nutritional status.

ADDRESSING THE IMPACT OF HIV AND AIDS ON THE YOUNG CHILD

The South African NIP for ECD (Departments of Education, Health, and Social Development, 2005, p. 12) states that

one of the aims of the NIP for ECD is to ensure access to an appropriate and effective integrated system of prevention, care and support services for children infected and affected by HIV and AIDS.

There are several different categories of child affected by HIV and AIDS in the community and the family (Foster, 2006). They include children who are infected; children living in households within which carers and/or other members have HIV or are already ill with AIDS related diseases (Brandt, 2007); children who have lost caregivers to AIDS (Richter et al., 2004); those who have been fostered by relatives or others; those in residential care; those living in child headed households; and a recently recognized category, those children who care for sick relatives and their siblings (Cluver & Gardiner, 2007).

Infants and children under five who are living with AIDS are extremely vulnerable. Most are likely to have been infected by vertical transmission, but older children may have been abused or infected on visits to clinical facilities through failures to observe protocols (Brookes, Shisana, & Richter, 2004). HIV also impacts on the neurological development of those who survive (Sher, 2005).

The focus of intervention with these children tends to be biomedical, through provision of antiretroviral medication and nutritional support. They are also more vulnerable to malnutrition, diarrhea, and pneumonia, and the risk of death is high. They present enormous challenges, particularly to caregivers in poor households who themselves are HIV positive and may be ill. In the first instance, prevention of mother to child transmission (PMTCT) is a priority. Apart from one province (the Western Cape), there is no reliable national data on the success of PMTCT programs. Antiretroviral treatment for infected children is a complex matter. Currently 36% of the estimated infected child population is on treatment, clearly very inadequate (Children's Rights Centre, 2009). A further crucial medical intervention is the provision of antiretroviral treatment for women. Currently 54% of eligible women receive treatment (Children's Rights Centre, 2009). The number with young children is not known. In this chapter we will not deal further with the specialized topic of the medical response to HIV positive children (see Saloojee, 2007), but instead we will focus on the social and psychological impacts that need to be addressed by interventions.

Richter and colleagues (2006) note that while children affected by AIDS face particular challenges, targeting this group is not helpful as there are children rendered vulnerable by factors other than AIDS in communities affected by the virus and

> such a large number of vulnerable children requires the urgent strengthening of systems to improve the situation of *all* children living in communities affected by HIV and AIDS—to complement programmes that support the most vulnerable children. (p. 9; emphasis added)

While needing to address the specific needs of children affected by HIV and AIDS, community-based programs should *not* contribute to the tendency to select these children out from among the many other vulnerable children in AIDS affected communities. Not only does this ignore the many other vulnerable children, it duplicates effort and results in stigma due to the justified jealously of those equally vulnerable who receive no support (Richter, Foster, and Sherr, 2006).

A key consideration is to support caregivers, particularly those who are ill. These women are at risk for depression, and as we have noted, this in turn increases the risk of child neglect due their lack of sensitivity to the child's needs caused by their own distress. The emerging evidence is that poor women on antiretrovirals are likely to have better well-being and less risk of depression than women with AIDS who are not (Brandt, 2007; Brandt et al., 2006). They would also benefit from psychosocial support (Cooper et al., 2009) coupled to psychosocial interventions designed to increase their sensitivity and responsiveness to their children. Initiatives to improve support from neighbors and other community members are also important.

In terms of interventions, South Africa does not have a developed evidence base on psychosocial interventions specifically for children who are living in households where caregivers have HIV and AIDS. In many respects this is not necessary as we can draw on the range of literature regarding the benefits of psychosocial support to vulnerable caregivers and households. In addition, Richter et al. (2006) point to the "naturally occurring" protective resources and to the importance of drawing upon them, particularly in countries and communities that do not have the benefit of the formal psychosocial programming:

> Psychosocial care and support is provided through interpersonal interactions that occur in caring relationships in everyday life, at home, school and in the community. This includes the love and protection that children experience in family environments, as well as interventions that assist children and families in coping. (pp. 14–15)

For these authors, *"psychosocial interventions"* and *"psychosocial support programming,"* interventions are distinguished from *"psychosocial care and support,"* which refers to the "everyday family systems of care which support children's psychosocial wellbeing" (p. 15). These everyday systems can of course be strengthened through intervention.

These are very useful distinctions that help us clarify what we mean when we talk about "psychosocial" interventions for young children affected by HIV and AIDS.

A key program message from Richter et al. (2006) is that

> children affected by HIV/AIDS have critical psychosocial needs. These are best addressed through supportive relationships and structures embedded in children's everyday lives. Standalone psychosocial interventions and programmes should *reinforce, and not replace, the essential psychosocial care and support that children receive from caregivers, relatives and friends*—support that occurs day-by-day and across the lifespan. (p. 29; emphasis added)

The first randomized controlled trial longitudinal study to be conducted in South Africa has recently appeared. The intervention tested the effects of a home visiting program that included an *early stimulation* component, on the neurodevelopmental status of young children infected with HIV. All the children were malnourished and their motor and cognitive development was delayed at baseline. The program was effective in improving the motor and cognitive outcomes of the children after a one year intervention. This is a very promising initiative.

Apart from this more recent research, Richter et al. (2006) note the dearth of good research on programming and stress the need for programs to be evaluated so that good practice can be established and programs can go to scale.

They list a range of promising responses to the situation of children affected by HIV and AIDS that is too detailed to reproduce here. To summarize, community and household level interventions for children living in family-like settings, the following are noted:

- home visits to monitor child well-being and raise awareness of children's needs; also to prevent abuse and provide support to vulnerable carers
- provision shelter and repair of shelter
- food support of various kinds
- a range of supports for access to health care particularly in rural areas
- provision of clothing to needy children
- availability of preschool programs (not necessarily formal)

- cash transfers
- specific support to families who foster orphans and other vulnerable children

Drawing on emerging evidence, Richter et al. (2006) provide a cogent argument for our need to support all vulnerable children in the family (or substitute family) context:

> The best way to support the wellbeing of young children affected by HIV/ AIDS is to strengthen and reinforce the circles of care that surround children. Children are best cared for by constant, committed and affectionate adults. When the caregiving circle is broken for some reason, extended families normally plug the gap. When the circle of care provided by kin is broken, community initiatives need to stand in, and when the circle of care provided by community is broken, external agencies need to play a part. Embracing all efforts should be a strong and continuous circle of support provided by government provision and legislative protection. The optimal use of the resources of external programmes is to assist communities in supporting families. Families are best placed to provide for the psychosocial needs of young children. When it is necessary for external agencies to provide direct services to children and to families, their touch should be light and, to be sustainable, it should be balanced by appropriate actions to strengthen extended family and community supports. (pp. 11–12)

These comments should alert us against the provision of residential care as far as possible except as an emergency resort. Expert opinion is strongly against this path (Foster, 2006; Richter et al., 2006). Residential care is more expensive, and particularly for infants and young children, long-term placement impacts negatively on a range child development outcomes in ways that cannot be reversed (Beckett et al., 2002; O'Connor et al., 2002). In addition, orphanages undermine traditional caregiving systems.

There has been a tendency in programming for children in communities affected by AIDS, to have a narrow psychological group and individual focus (e.g., bereavement work). While a limited number of children may need such intensive support, the vast majority will not. It is increasingly recognized that rather than these intensive program interventions, helping children to return to (or sustain) normal life functioning is crucial. This includes normalizing family functioning. As Richter et al. (2006) put it,

> Normalization involves helping a child feel safe in the context of their familiar surroundings and routines, receiving affection, nurturance and reassurance from supportive adults and older siblings, returning to school, and playing with friends. (p. 34)

And when traumatic events occur, such as the death of a parent, while care and support from familiar kin is essential rather than their becoming involved in quasi therapeutic sessions with unqualified people, "it is often best for young children's coping to be immersed in supportive day-to-day activities" (p. 35).

This section has not drawn on a strong randomized control trial or quasi experimental evidence base. They do not exist. Rather it links to what we know from tested interventions designed to support child development more generally in adverse circumstances. This knowledge has powerful relevance for this category of vulnerable children. Finally, early childhood centers can play a key role in provision of support to children affected by HIV and AIDS in their homes. South African initiatives seek to establish ECD sites as "nodes of support" for this group of children (Dawes, 2003). Affected children may face stigma and rejection from peers (and sometimes teachers). In poor households they may come to a preschool or community program without food; their progress may be affected by absences and poor concentration as a consequence of distress occasioned by losses, or their circumstances. There is no evidence as yet in South Africa for the success of interventions to support these children. However, the creation of caring early childhood environments would no doubt assist vulnerable children.

At the end of the day, *integrated* approaches that combine social, health, and material support to caregivers and families (and to schools and preschools) are needed to improve outcomes for young children affected by AIDS (Richter et al., 2006). The most effective way to do this is to strengthen the circle of care around the child wherever this occurs, whether this be the family, the school, or the clinical and social services.

CHILD MALTREATMENT PREVENTION

According to the World Health Organization and ISPCAN (2006, p. 7), child maltreatment "refers to the physical and emotional mistreatment, sexual abuse, neglect and negligent treatment of children, as well as to their commercial or other exploitation."

As we have indicated, children in South Africa are significantly at risk for exposure to violence, maltreatment and neglect. Child protection services can be conceptualized as being delivered at the four levels of intervention shown in Figure 2.2.

The figure is informed by the approach to child protection developed by the World Health Organization and ISPCAN (2006), and UNICEF's formulation of a Protective Environment. Service intensity and specialization

Figure 2.2
A hierarchy of interventions to improve child protection linked to the eight elements of the UNICEF Protective Environment

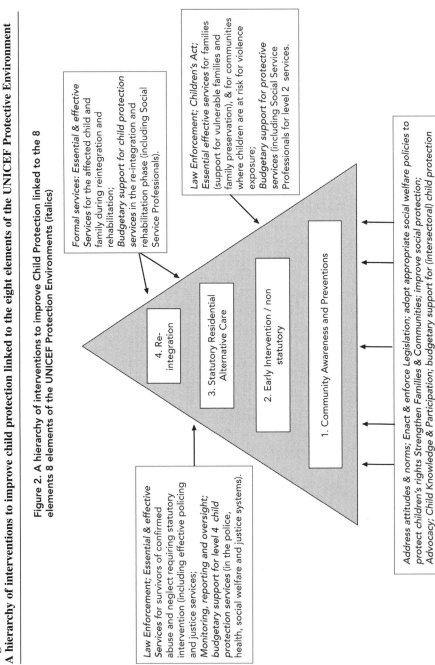

Figure 2. A hierarchy of interventions to improve Child Protection linked to the 8 elements 8 elements of the UNICEF Protection Environments (italics)

Formal services: Essential & effective Services for the affected child and family during reintegration and rehabilitation;
Budgetary support for child protection services in the re-integration and rehabilitation phase (including Social Service Professionals).

Law Enforcement; Children's Act;
Essential effective services for families (support for vulnerable families and family preservation), & for communities where children are at risk for violence exposure;
Budgetary support for protective services (including Social Service Professionals for level 2 services.

4. Re-integration

3. Statutory Residential Alternative Care

2. Early Intervention / non statutory

1. Community Awareness and Preventions

Law Enforcement; Essential & effective Services for survivors of confirmed abuse and neglect requiring statutory intervention (including effective policing and justice services;
Monitoring, reporting and oversight; budgetary support for level 4 child protection services (in the police, health, social welfare and justice systems).

Address attitudes & norms; Enact & enforce Legislation; adopt appropriate social welfare policies to protect children's rights Strengthen Families & Communities; improve social protection; Advocacy; Child Knowledge & Participation; budgetary support for (intersectoral) child protection increase as one moves toward the apex of the figure. This formulation is the basis of a Child Protection Plan developed for the Western Cape Province in South Africa developed by the first author of this chapter. It seeks to take account of very low service resources (less than half the social workers required for a minimal service) and an historic focus on services for children confirmed as maltreated.

The base of the pyramid includes initiatives to protect all children, the foundation being a policy and legislative framework that creates an environment in which the risk of exposure to violence, maltreatment, and abuse is reduced. The second level narrows the focus to interventions with children and families known to be at risk. At this level a key goal is to support vulnerable families and caregivers so as to inhibit family disintegration and reduce the risk that children will enter the formal child protection system (level 3 in Figure 2.2). Formal child protective services and reintegration form the highest levels of the service and are the most cost intensive (Barberton, 2006). As we have noted, South African and international evidence shows that young children are particularly vulnerable to maltreatment in the home (World Health Organization and ISP-CAN, 2006; Dawes & Ward, 2008). Level 2 in Figure 2.1 is a particularly important level at which to provide services if child maltreatment is to be prevented.

Intervention studies in developed regions of the world indicate that maltreatment can be reduced and prevented through interventions at levels 1 and 2 of the model in Figure 2.2, by using home visiting and parenting training, both of which have been and are currently being evaluated (Prinz, Sanders, Shapiro, Whitaker, & Lutzker, 2009; Sanders, 2003; Centers for Disease Control and Prevention, 2004).

Home visiting programs designed to improve maternal sensitivity and reduce intrusive and coercive maternal behaviors toward infants has been shown by Olds et al. (1998) reduce the risk of maltreatment. This program requires considerable investment and professional involvement that are likely to be well beyond the means of countries such as South Africa which have very significant numbers of parents living in conditions that raise the risk of maltreatment and neglect.

There is no South African data (and none from other African countries) on effective interventions to reduce the risk of maltreatment in vulnerable families.

However, the first randomized trial to test the efficacy of a home visiting program delivered to women living in poor urban households in Cape Town has proven to be effective in increasing maternal sensitivity and reducing intrusive interactions. In addition, more children in the trial showed secure attachment than controls as a result of the intervention (Cooper et al., 2009). While maltreatment prevention was not a goal of this trial, improvements in maternal sensitivity and related behaviors would be likely to reduce this risk. One of the most promising aspects of the South African trial is that it was delivered in 16 sessions by women from the same community as the target population who had no specialist trailing. This is a much more affordable approach and more appropriate as a preventive intervention for a country with limited resources than the approach of Olds et al. (1998). The program is now regularly delivered by a Cape Town NGO, the Parent Center (http://www.parentcentre.org.za/), and is designed to operate at level 2 in Figure 2.1. It remains to be seen, however, whether an intervention such as the Cape Town trial would be efficacious in multiproblem families in which maltreatment has already been identified or appears to be a serious risk.

A pioneering South African program, the Perinatal Mental Health Project at the University of Cape Town, provides counseling support to depressed women in poor communities prior to and after giving birth (http://www.psychiatry.uct.ac.za/pmhp/). By the end of 2008, more than 5,000 pregnant women had been offered antenatal screening for psychological distress. Of those screened, 33% qualified for referral. Counseling services are provided to deal with problems ranging from the need for primary support such as social grants, to depression and other psychological problems. Clients attend two to three sessions on average and a limited postnatal follow-up is provided. The program remains to be evaluated, and measures of parent–child interaction are not currently undertaken. However, programs of this nature have the potential to deliver cost-effective preventive mental health services that benefit the mother, and which have the secondary effect of reducing the risk of poor early mother–child relationships that may be precursors of harsh, neglectful, or abusive parenting.

PROGRAMMING FOR EARLY CHILDHOOD COGNITIVE DEVELOPMENT IN THE YEARS BEFORE SCHOOL

Reviews of the available evidence indicate that the most effective interventions to improve young child development outcomes in vulnerable populations are those that are comprehensive and deliver a package of services such as nutrition, health care, parenting support, and direct child stimulation (e.g., Grantham-McGregor et al., 2007; Dawes, Biersteker, & Irvine,

2008). In this section we consider South African initiatives aimed at improving child cognitive outcomes with the aim of facilitating progress in the schooling system and building the basis for skilled participation in the labor market. However, the success of these will depend to a great extent on other services for children also being in place.

Provision of early childhood education services in South Africa is available through programs delivered directly to children in reception year classes and community-based ECD centers as well as through a small but growing number of home-based and community-based programs that focus on training parents to provide stimulation experiences that prepare children for the schooling system.

Increasing access and quality of center-based ECD services for under fives has received high level political recognition and increased budget resources over the last five years. This is largely based on arguments that draw a link between schooling outcomes and increased productivity in adulthood drawing on evidence from very well resourced interventions in North America. There is very little evidence on the impact of South African ECD programs. Only two small-scale unpublished outcome studies are available for South African formal ECD evaluations. The programs evaluated were NGO run and had a great deal of professional support as well as favorable teacher child ratios. Both found gains in child outcomes relevant to schooling following participation in high-quality, center-based programs compared with control groups (Herbst, 1996; Vinjevold, 1996). Short and Biersteker (1984) followed the scholastic performance of ECD center participants into adolescence and they performed above the average in their school population. There are no peer-reviewed studies (Biersteker & Dawes, 2008).

Efforts to improve the quality of ECD center draw on the accepted quality indicators in international practice, there is a focus on increasing the number of registered programs in order to ensure adherence to minimum norms and standards including parent involvement and an extensive public funded training program has been put in place to improve educational qualifications of practitioners. This goes hand in hand with a program to increase subsidies on a poverty targeted basis. A recent study of center quality however, indicates that these interventions are insufficient to guarantee more than a minimum level of care and stimulation (Department of Social Development Western Cape, 2010). The need for regular and appropriate on-site monitoring and support as well as attention to wages and service conditions for staff has been identified in several studies (e.g., Biersteker, 2008, 2009; Moll, 2007; Department of Social Development Western Cape, 2010).

Through the NIP for ECD (Departments of Education, Health, and Social Development, 2005) government has recognized that most young children will not attend an ECD center and announced a policy intention to support caregivers to provide stimulation at home and in informal community provision such as playgroups and parenting education programs. There are many examples of such programs in South Africa but while there is ample evidence that they can improve young children's access to health and social services and are valued by parents and other primary caregivers their impact on psychosocial outcomes has not yet been evaluated.

The international evidence base suggests that a number of essential conditions for improving psychosocial outcomes include two generational interventions (parent and child) over at least a year and on a frequent (at least weekly) and delivered by practitioners who are trained in appropriate skills for working with parents (Dawes et al., 2008; Evans, 2007). A rapid assessment and analysis of home- and community-based programs in South Africa (Biersteker, 2007) indicated that support to families was not offered as frequently or for as long as in successful programs in other countries. For example the Department of Social Development has developed a training package for an 11-session capacity building parents/primary caregivers to support young child development (Department of Social Development, 2008). A number of trainers located in NGOs and ECD representative structures were trained with the intention that they will in turn cascade this program and use it flexibly for their different constituencies as weekly sessions or as a block of training.

A first South African initiative to rigorously test the effects of different home- and center-based interventions on child cognitive and language outcomes as well as on service linkages and changes in the care environment began in 2008 and will be completed in 2011 (Dawes & Biersteker, 2009). Five NGOs have each developed an integrated area-based strategy. Components include the following:

- **Home-based programs** in changing parenting and other aspects of caregiver behavior that are associated with improvements in children's nutrition, protection, and development—in particular: motor, language, cognition, and socioemotional domains, and that link families to services for the benefit of the child
- **Center enrichment programs** (preschool and grade R) in improving site functioning, teacher practice, and children's psychological development; and in linking families to services (these interventions include governing body training)

- **Playgroup interventions** for children not in formal ECD in improving children's developmental outcomes and linking families to services
- **Advocacy** interventions with provincial and local authorities to improve access to services for the young child
- **School transition programs** that enable schools to be prepared for young children and for young children and families to be familiarized with the transition to school

CONCLUSIONS

South Africa is a middle income but very unequal society. More than 60% of children fall within the poorest 40% of the population. The risks to sound early child development and mental health are significant with the most important being the broad impact of poverty environments with associated malnutrition, HIV and AIDS (in both caregivers and young children), neglect and maltreatment, and an early environment that fails to provide the majority of children with the necessary learning and stimulation to prepare the child for school. As the majority will never be able to afford a preschool, home-based initiatives to improve the quality of care and stimulation received by the child are necessary. We still need to establish the most efficacious and cost-effective way to deliver such programs to scale.

Early preventive intervention in each of these areas is crucial if a sound platform for life is to be established, and it is essential that governments in countries such as South Africa commit significant resources to improving the situation of young children. The long-term returns on investment in the early years for human capital development have been amply demonstrated (Heckman, 2006).

NOTES

1. All figures provided by Statistics South Africa (http://www.statssa. gov.za/).

2. During the apartheid period prior to 1994, South Africans were classified as either white, black (belonging to an indigenous African ethnic group), colored (mixed-race descent), or Indian (descendents of indentured laborers brought from the Indian subcontinent during the late 19th and early 20th centuries). While these categories are still used in official statistics, we reject them as racist. For present purposes, we disaggregate in white and black (all three categories of persons of color).

3. The Gini coefficient is based on the income distribution and ranges in value from 0 (equality) to 1 (inequality).

REFERENCES

Aber, J. L., & Bennett, N. G. (1997). The effects of poverty on child health and development. *Annual Review of Public Health, 18,* 463–483.

ACC/SCN. (1997). Stunting and young child development. In *The third report on the world nutrition situation.* Geneva, Switzerland: Author. Retrieved from http://www.unsystem.org/scn/archives/rwns03/index.htm

Barberton, C. (2006). *The cost of the Children's Bill—estimates of the cost to government of the services envisaged by the Comprehensive Children's Bill for the period 2005 to 2010.* Pretoria, South Africa: Department of Social Development.

Beckett, C., Bredenkamp, D., Bredenkamp, D., Castle, J., Groothues, C., O'Connor, T. G., et al. (2002). Behaviour patterns associated with institutional deprivation: A study of children adopted from Romania. *Journal of Developmental & Behavioral Pediatrics, 23,* 297–303.

Biersteker, L. (2007). *Rapid assessment and analysis of innovative community and home-based childminding and ECD programmes in support of poor and vulnerable babies and young children in South Africa.* Pretoria, South Africa: UNICEF.

Biersteker, L. (2008). *Towards a job hierarchy for ECD provision and supervision in South Africa, and the fit of low-skill service providers scaling up early childhood development (0–4 years) in South Africa.* Cape Town: Human Sciences Research Council.

Biersteker, L. (2009). Introducing a reception year (grade R) for children aged five years as a first year of schooling. Washington, DC: Brookings Institute Wolfensohn Center Early Child Development Project.

Biersteker, L., & Dawes, A. (2008). Early childhood development. In A. Kraak (Ed.), *HRD review 2008 education, employment and skills* (pp. 186–205). Cape Town: HSRC Press.

Biersteker, L., & Kvalsvig, J. (2007). Early childhood development and the home-care environment in the pre-school years. In A. Dawes, R. Bray, & A. Van der Merwe (Eds.), *Monitoring child wellbeing: A South African rights-based approach* (pp. 159–190). Cape Town: HSRC Press.

Black, M. M., Baqui, A. H., Zaman, K., McNary, S. W., Hamadani, J. D., Parveen, M., et al. (2007). Depressive symptoms among rural Bangladeshi mothers: implications for infant development. *Journal of Child Psychology and Psychiatry, 48,* 764–772.

Bradshaw, D., Bourne, D., & Nannan, N. (2003). *MRC policy brief: What are the leading causes of death among South African children?* Tygerberg, South Africa: Medical Research Council.

Brandt, R. (2007). Does HIV matter when you are poor and how? The impact of HIV/AIDS on the psychological adjustment of South African mothers in the era of HAART (Unpublished doctoral dissertation). University of Cape Town, South Africa.

Brandt, R., Dawes, A., & Bray, R. (2006). Women coping with AIDS in Africa: Contributions of a contextually grounded research methodology. *Psychology, Health & Medicine, 11*, 522–527.

Bray, R., & Brandt, R. (2007). Child care and poverty in South Africa: An ethnographic challenge to conventional interpretations. *Journal of Children and Poverty, 13*, 1–19.

Brookes, H., Shisana, O., & Richter, L. M. (2004). *The national household HIV prevalence and risk survey of South African Children.* Cape Town: HSRC Publishers.

Budlender, D. (2008). *Feasibility and appropriateness of attaching behavioural conditions to a social support grant for children aged 15–17 years.* Pretoria, South Africa: Department of Social Development.

Cawson, P., Wattam, C., Brooker, S., & Kelly, C. (2000). *Child maltreatment in the United Kingdom: A study of the prevalence of child abuse and neglect.* London: National Society for the Prevention of Cruelty to Children.

Centers for Disease Control and Prevention. (2004). *Using evidence-based parenting programs to advance CDC efforts in child maltreatment prevention.* Retrieved from http://www.cdc.gov/ncipc/pub-res/parenting/ChildMalT-Briefing.pdf.

Children's Rights Centre. (2009). *Scorecard 2009: Weighing up South Africa's response to children and HIV and AIDS.* Durban: Children's Rights Centre. Retrieved from http://www.crc-sa.co.za/.

Cluver, L., & Gardner, F. (2007). Risk and protective factors for psychological well-being of orphaned children in Cape Town: A qualitative study of children's views. *AIDS Care, 19*(3), 318–325.

Cluver, L., Gardner, F., & Operario, D. (2007). Psychological distress amongst AIDS-orphaned children in urban South Africa. *Journal of Child Psychology and Psychiatry, 48*(8), 755–763.

Cooper, P. J., Tomlinson, M., Swartz, L., Landman, M., Molteno, C., Stein, A., et al. (2009). Improving the quality of the mother–infant relationship and infant attachment in a socio-economically deprived community in a South African context: A randomised controlled trial. *British Medical Journal, 338,* b974. doi:10.1136/bmj.b974

Couper, J. (2002). Prevalence of childhood disability in rural KwaZulu-Natal. *South African Medical Journal, 92,* 549–552.

Dawes, A. (2003). Improving school children's mental health in an era of HIV/AIDS. In M. Taylor & J. D. Kvalsvig (Eds.), *Colloquium report: Improving the health of school age children in an era of HIV/AIDS—Linking policies, programmes and strategies for the 21st century.* Department of Community Health, Nelson Mandela School of Medicine, University of Natal, and the Child, Youth, and Family Development Programme. Durban, South Africa: Human Sciences Research Council.

Dawes, A., & Biersteker, L. (2009, July). Improving the quality of ECD interventions through results-based monitoring and evaluation: The

Sobambisana initiative. Paper presented at the Pan-African ECD Conference, Johannesburg.

Dawes, A., Biersteker, L., & Irvine, M. (2008). *What makes a difference to child outcomes in the period 0–4? Inputs for quality ECD interventions—Scaling up early childhood development (0–4 years) in South Africa.* Cape Town: Human Sciences Research Council.

Dawes, A., & Mushwana, M. (2007). Child abuse and neglect. In A. Dawes, R. Bray, & A. Van der Merwe (Eds.), *Monitoring child wellbeing: A South African rights-based approach* (pp. 269–292). Cape Town: HSRC Press.

Dawes, A., & Ward, C. L. (2008). Levels, trends, and determinants of child maltreatment in the Western Cape Province. In R. Marindo (Ed.), *The state of population in the Western Cape Province* (pp. 97–205). Cape Town: HSRC Press.

Dawes, A., de Sas Kropiwnicki, Z., Kafaar, Z., & Richter, L. (2006). Partner violence. In U. Pillay, B. Roberts, & S. Rule (Eds.), *South African social attitudes: Changing times, diverse voices* (pp. 225–251). Cape Town: HSRC Press.

Department of Education. (2001). *Early childhood development* (White Paper No. 5). Pretoria, South Africa: Author.

Department of Education. (2008). *2007 grade 3 systemic evaluation leaflet.* Retrieved from http://www.doe.gov.za/.

Department of Social Development. (2008). *Parental/primary caregiver capacity building training package.* Pretoria, South Africa: Author/UNICEF.

Department of Social Development Western Cape. (2010). *Western Cape Department of Social Development 2009 audit of early childhood development facility quality.* Cape Town: Author.

Departments of Education, Health, and Social Development. (2005). *National Integrated Plan for Early Childhood Development in South Africa 2005–2010.* Pretoria, South Africa: Author.

Engel, P. L., Black, M. M., Behrman, J. R., Cabral de Mello, M., Gertler, P. J., Kapiriri, L., et al. (2007). Strategies to avoid the loss of developmental potential in more than 200 million children in the developing world. *The Lancet, 369,* 229–242.

Evans, E. (2007). *Parenting programmes an important ECD intervention strategy.* Background paper prepared for the Education for All Global Monitoring Report 2007 Strong Foundations: Early Childhood Care and Education, Paris, UNESCO.

Fieggen, G., Wiemann, M., Brown, C., Van As, S., Swingler, G., & Peter, J. (2004). Inhuman shields: Children caught in the crossfire of domestic violence. *South African Medical Journal, 94,* 293–296.

Finkelhor, D. (2008). *Childhood victimisation: Violence, crime, and abuse in the lives of young people.* Oxford: Oxford University Press.

Flisher, A. J., Dawes, A., Kafaar, Z., Lund, C., Sorsdahl, C., Myers, B., et al. (in press). Child and adolescent mental health in South Africa. In E. Akyeampong,

A. Hill, and A. Kleinman (Eds.), *Psychiatry in Africa*. Bloomington: Indiana University Press.

Foster, G. (2006). Children who live in communities affected by AIDS. *The Lancet, 367*, 700–701.

Garcia, M., Pence, A., & Evans, J. L. (Eds.). (2008). *Africa's future, Africa's challenge: Early childhood care and development in Sub-Saharan Africa*. Washington, DC: World Bank.

Grantham-McGregor, S., Cheung, Y. B., Cueto, S., Glewwe, P., Richter, L., & Strupp, B. (2007). Developmental potential in the first 5 years for children in developing countries. *The Lancet, 369*, 60–70.

Heckman, J. J. (2006). Skill formation and the economics of investing in disadvantaged children. *Science, 312*, 1900–1902.

Hendricks, M., Eley, B., & Bourne, L. (2006). Child nutrition. In P. Ijumba & A. Padarath (Eds.), *South African health review 2006* (pp. 203–220). Durban: Health Systems Trust.

Herbst, I. (1996). Evaluation of the effects of Ntataise Early Childhood Stimulation Project. Unpublished report prepared for the Joint Education Trust.

Jewkes, R., Levin, J., & Penn-Kekana, L. (2002). Risk factors for domestic violence: Findings from a South African cross-sectional study. *Social Science & Medicine, 55*, 1603–1617.

Kleintjies, S., Flisher, A. J., Fick, M., Railoun, A., Lund, C., Molteno, C. D., et al. (2006). The prevalence of mental disorders among children, adolescents and adults in the Western Cape, South Africa. *South African Psychiatry Review, 9*, 157–160.

Kruger, H. S., Swart, R., Labadarios, D., Dannhauser, A., & Nel, J. H. (2007). Anthropometric status. In D. Labadarios (Ed.), *National Food Consumption Survey Fortification Baseline, South Africa 2005* (pp. 121–160). Pretoria, South Africa: Directorate Nutrition, Department of Health.

Le Roux, K. (2006). *Predictors of speed of rehabilitation of malnourished children in a home based community outreach nutrition programme in a township outside Cape Town, South Africa* (Degree Project Research Series 2006 No. 1). Uppsala, Sweden: Department of Women and Child Health, Uppsala University.

Lewin, S., Dick, J., Pond, P., Zwarenstein, M., Aja, G. N., vanWyk, B. E., et al. (2005). Lay health workers in primary and community health care. *Cochrane Database of Systematic Reviews, 1*. Retrieved from CD004015.DOI: 10.1002/14651858.CD004015.pub2.

Martorell, R. (1996, April). Under-nutrition during pregnancy and early childhood and its consequences for behavioral development. Paper for discussion at the World Bank's conference Early Child Development: Investing in the Future, Carter Center of Emory University, Atlanta, GA.

Moll, I. (2007). *The state of grade R provision in South Africa and recommendations for priority interventions within it*. Braamfontein: SAIDE.

Naidoo, S. (2000). A profile of the oro-facial injuries in child physical abuse at a children's hospital. *Child Abuse & Neglect, 24*, 521–534.

O'Connor, T. G., Rutter, M., Beckett, C., Keaveney, L., Kreppner, J., & English and Romanian Adoptees Study Team. (2002). The effects of global severe privation on cognitive competence: Extension and longitudinal follow-up. *Child Development, 71*, 376–390.

Olds, D., Henderson, C. J., Kitzman, H., Eckenrode, J., Cole, R., & Tatelbaum, R. (1998). The promise of home visitation: Results of two randomized trials. *Journal of Community Psychology, 26*, 5–21.

Pelletier, D. L. (1994). The relationship between child anthropometry and mortality in developing countries: Implications for policy—Programs and future research. *Journal of Nutrition, 124*(Suppl.), S2047–S2081.

Potterton, J. L., & Baillieu, N. (2008). The extent of delay of language, motor, and cognitive development in HIV-positive infants. *Journal of Neurologic Physical Therapy, 32*, 118–121.

Prinz, R. J., Sanders, M. R., Shapiro, C. J., Whitaker, D. J., & Lutzker, J. R. (2009). Population-based prevention of child maltreatment: The U.S. Triple P System population trial. *Prevention Science, 10*, 1–12.

Rehle, T., Shisana, T., Pillay, V., Zuma, K., Puren, A., & Parker, W. (2007). National HIV incidence measures—new insights into the South African epidemic. *South African Medical Journal, 97*, 194–199.

Republic of South Africa. (2009). *Development indicators 2009*. Pretoria, South Africa: Presidency.

Richter, L. M. (1994). Economic stress and its influence on the family and caretaking patterns. In A. Dawes & D. Donald (Eds.), *Childhood and adversity: Psychological perspectives from South African research* (pp. 28–48). Cape Town: David Philip Publishers.

Richter, L. M. (2004). *Early child development in resource poor settings: Balancing children's material and mental needs*. Geneva: World Health Organization. Retrieved from http://www.who.int/child-adolescent-health/publications/CHILD_HEALTH/ISBN_92_4_159134_X.htm.

Richter, L. M., & Dawes, A. (2008). Child abuse in South Africa: Rights and wrongs. *Child Abuse Review, 17*(2), 79–93.

Richter, L. M., Foster, G., & Sherr, L. (2006). *Where the heart is: Meeting the psychosocial needs of young children in the context of HIV/AIDS*. The Hague: Bernard van Leer Foundation.

Richter, L. M., & Grieve, K. W. (1991). Home environment and cognitive development of black infants in impoverished South African families. *Infant Mental Health Journal, 12*, 88–102.

Richter, L. M., Manegold, J., & Pather, R. (2004). *Family and community interventions for children affected by AIDS*. Cape Town: Human Sciences Research Council.

Saloojee, H. (2007). Monitoring child health. In A. Dawes, R. Bray, & A. Van der Merwe (Eds.), *Monitoring child well-being: A South African rights-based approach* (pp. 93–109). Cape Town: HSRC Press.

Schneider, M., & Saloojee, G. (2007). Monitoring childhood disability. In A. Dawes, R. Bray, & A. Van der Merwe (Eds.), *Monitoring child well-being: A*

South African rights-based approach (pp. 191–212). Cape Town: HSRC Press.

Sher, L. (2005). *Young children and HIV/AIDS, mapping the field* (Working Papers in ECD, Young Children and HIV/AIDS Subseries No. 33). The Hague: Van Leer Foundation.

Shisana, O., Rehle, T., Simbayi, L. C., Parker, W., Zuma, K., Bhana, A., et al. (2005). *South African national HIV prevalence, HIV incidence, behaviour and communications survey.* Cape Town: HSRC Press.

Short, A., & Biersteker, L. (1984). *Evaluation of the Early Learning Centre centre-based programmes with follow-up through adolescence.* Athlone, Cape Town: Early Learning Resource Unit.

Statistics South Africa. (1999). *Thematic report on children based on Census '96.* Pretoria, South Africa: Author.

Statistics South Africa. (2007). *The coverage and quality of birth registration data in South Africa, 1998–2005.* Report No. 03-06-01. Pretoria, South Africa: Author.

Statistics South Africa. (2009a). *Mid-year population estimates 2009* (Statistical Release No. P0302). Pretoria, South Africa: Author.

Statistics South Africa. (2009b). *General Household Survey 2008* (Statistical Release No. P0318). Pretoria, South Africa: Author.

Streak, J., Yu, D., & van der Berg, D. (2008). Measuring child poverty in South Africa. *HSRC Review, 6*(4), 33–34.

Swart, R., Sanders, D., & McLachlan, M. (2008). Nutrition: A primary health care perspective. In P. Barron & J. Roma-Reardon (Eds.), *South African health review 2008* (pp. 129–148). Durban, South Africa: Health Systems Trust.

Tomlinson, M., Cooper, P. J., Stein, A., Swartz, L., & Molteno, C. (2006). Post-partum depression and infant growth in a South African peri-urban settlement. *Child Care, Health and Development, 32,* 81–86.

Vinjevold, P. (1996). Evaluation of the impact of ECD programmes. *Joint Education Trust Bulletin, 3,* 5–7.

Walker, S. P., Chang, S. M., Powell, C. A., & Grantham-McGregor, S. M. (2005). Effects of early childhood psychosocial stimulation and nutritional supplementation on cognition and education in growth-stunted Jamaican children: Prospective cohort study. *The Lancet, 366,* 1804–1807.

Walker, S. P., Wachs, T. D., Meeks Gardner, J., Lozoff, B., Wasserman, G. A., Pollitt, E., et al. (2007). Child development: Risk factors for adverse outcomes in developing countries. *The Lancet, 369,* 145–157.

World Health Organization & ISPCAN. (2006). *Preventing child maltreatment: A guide to taking action and generating evidence.* Geneva, Switzerland: Author.

Young, M. E., & Mustard, J. F. (2008). Brain development and ECD. In M. Garcia, A. Pence, & J. L. Evans (Eds.), *Africa's future, Africa's challenge: Early childhood care and development in Sub-Saharan Africa* (pp. 71–113). Washington, DC: World Bank.

Chapter 3

A FAMILY DISEASE: MENTAL HEALTH OF CHILDREN ORPHANED BY AIDS AND LIVING WITH HIV+ CAREGIVERS

Lucie Cluver, Don Operario, Frances Gardner, and Mark E. Boyes

HIV/AIDS is a family disease. It impacts *all* members of the nuclear and extended family emotionally, financially, and through the pervasive stigma which accompanies HIV infection. Much of the care and responsibility for AIDS-affected people, and for their children, rests within the wider family. Families are also the focus of efforts to find solutions for the care of children who are infected or affected by HIV/AIDS. This chapter examines the mental health of parents and children living in HIV-infected families. We will focus on two main regions: sub-Saharan Africa and the United States. This is because (1) the great majority of available evidence comes from these two regions, and (2) these two regions are affected by the same disease but represent very different epidemics in very different social contexts. However, it is to be noted that the number of studies in the United States remains very small, and so comparisons between regions should be treated with caution.

In sub-Saharan Africa, HIV is largely transmitted through heterosexual contact, often within marriage (Hudson, 1996). Theories that aim to explain the massive spread of the epidemic in sub-Saharan Africa emphasize the effects of societal factors including labor migration, poverty, and gender inequality (Dunkle et al., 2004), which exacerbate behavioral and biomedical factors associated with HIV transmission. HIV prevalence rates for women in sub-Saharan antenatal clinics range from 12% in Zimbabwe to nearly 40% in Swaziland, and overall prevalence rates in adult populations (15- to 49-year-olds) are as high as 26% (see Table 3.1) (UNAIDS, 2008).

Table 3.1
Number of people living with HIV/AIDS and adult prevalence rates in a sample of sub-Saharan African countries

Country	People living with HIV/AIDS	Adult (15–49) prevalence
Botswana	300,000	23.9%
Kenya	1.5 to 2 million	7.1% to 8.5%
Lesotho	270,000	23.2%
Malawi	930,000	11.9%
Nigeria	2.6 million	3.1%
South Africa	5.7 million	18.1%
Swaziland	190,000	26.1%
Uganda	1 million	6.7%
Zambia	1.1 million	15.2%
Zimbabwe	1.3 million	15.3%

Note: Statistics taken from UNAIDS (2008) report on the global AIDS epidemic.

In South Africa, as in many other countries, black African and other impoverished groups are most severely affected by HIV.

In the United States, the heterosexual epidemic again disproportionately affects specific ethnic groups, in particular African Americans and Latinos (Centers for Disease Control and Prevention, 2007). For example, in 2005 approximately 64% of all females living with HIV/AIDS in the United States were African American (Centers for Disease Control and Prevention, 2007). However, while heterosexual transmission remains a source of infection, other major sources of infection include transmission between men who have sex with men (MSM) (Centers for Disease Control and Prevention, 2007, 2009), intravenous drug use (Des Jarlais et al., 2005), and forced sex in prison (Springer & Altice, 2005). This means that many families in the United States are coping not only with HIV infection but also with a range of other associated social problems.

As of 2008, an estimated 20 million children worldwide had lost a parent to HIV/AIDS, and even with the expansion of antiretroviral treatment access by 2015 the number of orphaned children will still be overwhelmingly high. The vast majority of these children (approximately 12 million) live in sub-Saharan Africa (UNAIDS, 2008). In South Africa alone, 3.4 million children are parentally bereaved, with around 65% of deaths attributable to HIV/AIDS (Anderson & Phillips, 2006). In areas where antiretroviral treatment (ART; or highly active antiretroviral treatment,

HAART) is available and accessible, parents are surviving longer and many are able to survive until their children reach adulthood. Far less is known about numbers of children who are living with an HIV+ parent or caregiver. To the best of our knowledge there are no available data revealing proportions of HIV-infected people who care for children, or the number of children living in HIV-affected families. We can estimate that these numbers are in the millions in countries with generalized epidemics, but further research is essential in order to identify this potentially vulnerable group. We also know very little about the proportion of children living with caregivers who are on ART medication, or the benefits for the health and well-being of these children, compared with those living with caregivers who are not.

Most children living with an HIV+ parent or caregiver are not themselves HIV+; however, a significant proportion of these children are. About 17% of new HIV infections annually are in children of up to 14 years of age (UNAIDS, 2008). Pooled analyses of data in sub-Saharan Africa studies indicate most of these infections occur through vertical transmission (Newell et al., 2004), although findings from South Africa highlight other routes of transmission including sexual abuse and infection in health facilities (Brookes, Shishana, & Richter, 2004). Importantly, research suggests that children who are HIV infected may experience distinct cognitive difficulties and mental health issues (Mellins, Brackis-Cott, Abrams, & Dolezal, 2006; Mellins et al., 2009), in addition to the effects of having an HIV+ or deceased parent. Additionally, the demographics of this group differ between countries in which antiretroviral treatment has been available at different times. For example, the United States has provided ART to perinatally infected infants since the mid-1990s (Havens, Mellins, & Hunter, 2002) and now has a cohort of HIV+ adolescents who are approaching adulthood (Bush-Parker, 2000). In contrast, Botswana began providing pediatric ART in January 2002, while South Africa only published a plan to provide pediatric ART in the public health care system in late 2003.

This chapter explores the evidence suggesting that familial HIV sickness and death impacts negatively on the mental health and well-being of both parents and children. Additionally, we briefly discuss the implications of this research for intervention strategies targeting children's needs. A broad framework that informs much of this chapter is Bronfenbrenner's ecological model (Bronfenbrenner, 1979). This model puts children at the center of multiple, interacting layers of influence (see Figure 3.1). Proximal to the child are relationships with caregivers and the everyday caregiving environment. More distal are school and community influences,

Figure 3.1
"Circles of care," an adaptation of Bronfenbrenner's ecological model

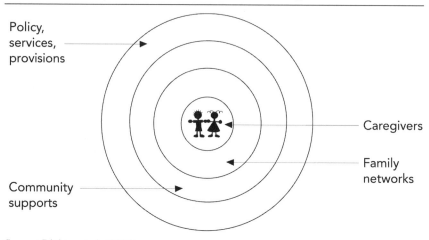

Source: Richter et al. (2006).

followed by wider political, policy, and cultural factors, which determine the context of child development. Key to this theoretical framework, and supported by research on risk and resilience (Luthar, Cicchetti, & Becker, 2000; Rutter, 2006), is the cumulative and counterbalancing effects of these risk and protective factors acting on each other, and on the child, as well as the effects of the child's initiatives acting on his or her external environment. From this perspective, the impacts of adversity in particular spheres of a child's life can be mitigated by positive factors in another sphere (Bronfenbrenner, 1979). Thus, while HIV is a family disease, it also necessitates a family response. Not only does the infection of one family member have multiple and long-term effects on all other family members, but it is also clear that the family are the primary source of care and support for AIDS-affected children. For children where family are unavailable, unwilling, or unable to provide care, support groups within the wider communities may need strengthening and support in sustaining care for HIV/AIDS-affected children.

MENTAL HEALTH IMPACTS

Any sickness or death within a family can have an impact on children's mental health and well-being. Studies of children whose mothers have cancer reveal that these children often experience emotional and behavioral difficulties, as well as fears of parental death (Forrest, Plumb,

Ziebland, & Stein, 2006). In 2000, a review of the impact of parental death on mental health (although this review did not include HIV-related death) reported that emotional problems may manifest differently according to developmental age (Dowdney, 2000); for example bedwetting among younger children and depression and guilt among adolescents (Dowdney et al., 1999). This review also reported more internalizing problems (such as depression) among bereaved girls, while more externalizing (behavior) problems were reported among bereaved boys. Children's mental health is especially at risk in the context of traumatic parental death, such as suicide (Dowdney, 2000) or homicide (Black & Harris-Hendricks, 1992). Importantly, until the late 1990s, the vast majority of literature on child mental health in the context of parental illness or death was Western-focused and did not yet address AIDS-related death. However, the rapid spread of HIV and the subsequent rise in numbers of AIDS orphans has led to a new body of evidence, clustered in sub-Saharan Africa and the United States. In order to understand how familial HIV can affect childhood mental health, it is important to look at impacts on both the infected person in their caregiving role and on children themselves.

HIV/AIDS, Parents, and Parenting

There is strong evidence suggesting that children's emotional well-being is closely connected to that of their parent or caregiver (Cluver, Gardner, & Operario, 2009; Stein, Ramchandani, & Murray, 2008). In Africa most HIV+ women are diagnosed during pregnancy. In rural South Africa women coming to terms with a serious illness report experiencing emotions of shock, grief, and fear, as well as motivational dilemmas regarding the unborn child (whom the parent is at risk of infecting) (Rochat et al., 2006). Enduring emotional problems have also been reported in HIV-infected mothers of young children in urban South Africa (Brandt, 2009). Similarly, high levels of depression and anxiety among HIV+ parents of adolescents have also been reported in the United States (Rotheram-Borus, Lightfoot, & Shen, 1999).

HIV infection can cause cognitive problems, even at early stages. At later stages of AIDS illness, people can experience severe mental illnesses such as AIDS-related dementia or psychotic symptoms (Antinori et al., 2007). These AIDS-related cognitive impairments or feelings of depression and anxiety may for some people impact on parenting. Additionally, for parents who have become infected through injection drug use or in prison (more likely to occur in the United States than in sub-Saharan Africa), there are likely to be other emotional and behavioral problems that can also affect children in their care. Parenting may also be made more difficult due to the stigma associated with HIV. The ongoing stigma of infection can reduce support systems, and HIV-infected parents also report ostracism and stigma when trying to access health care for themselves and their children (Green & Smith, 2004). Moreover, as parents experience increasing numbers of opportunistic infections, their own physical health problems can impact on parenting capacity. In addition, many HIV-infected caregivers are also caring for other infected family members, such as spouses, siblings, or children. Studies have revealed that parents are often preoccupied with worries about their and their children's HIV infection and health (Simoni, Davis, Drossman, & Weinberg, 2000). Finally, HIV/AIDS places incredible financial pressure on many families and poverty has been shown to impact on parenting, especially under stressful conditions (Aber, Jones, & Raver, 2007). Even where health care is free, AIDS illness often results in loss of earnings, and in sub-Saharan Africa the costs of AIDS treatment and funerals frequently result in deficits in children's nutrition and education (Booysen, 2002; Case & Ardington, 2005). While parenting is often a challenging experience, parenting with HIV (and in the contexts of stigma and poverty) may be even harder.

Orphaned Children

There is strong and remarkably consistent evidence (from both the United States and sub-Saharan Africa) that AIDS orphanhood impacts negatively on mental health and well-being. Contrary to early fears that orphans may be "unsocialized" and "potential rebels" (Barnett & Whiteside, 2002; Hunter, 1990), there is little empirical evidence of severe behavioral problems. However, multiple studies from sub-Saharan Africa reveal that AIDS orphanhood is associated with increased levels of emotional distress, particularly depression, anxiety and posttraumatic stress (see Figure 3.2 for an example) (Atwine, Cantor-Graae, & Bajunirwe, 2005; Bhargava, 2005; Cluver, Gardner, & Operario, 2007; Forehand et al., 1999; Makame, Ani, & McGregor, 2002; Nyamukapa et al., 2008). Recent data from China suggest similar emotional distress in Chinese AIDS orphans, but as yet these data lack comparisons with nonorphaned groups (Zhao et al., 2007). Furthermore, mental health impacts are not restricted to AIDS orphans. A recent large study and systematic review investigated caregivers of orphaned children (mainly grandparents) and found that these caregivers also reported heightened levels of depression and anxiety (Kuo & Operario, 2009a, 2009b). Similarly, qualitative studies have also reported

Figure 3.2
Proportions of children in range for clinical-level disorder in South Africa

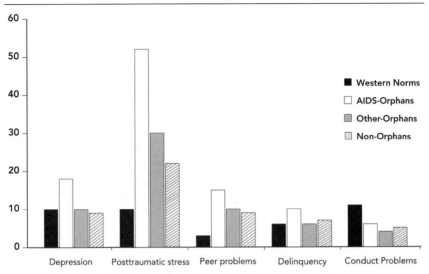

Source: Cluver et al. (2007).

heightened distress among grandmothers caring for orphaned children, while also grieving for the death of their adult child (Ferreira, Keikelame, & Mosaval, 2001). Studies conducted in the United States report similar findings to those in Africa, although with additional evidence of behavioral problems among children with HIV+ parents (Forehand et al., 2002; Rotheram-Borus, Lee, Lin, & Lester, 2004). However, the extent to which these behavioral problems may be connected to other social problems in HIV-infected families in the United States—such as increased likelihood for poverty, parental incarceration, and parental substance use—is not known and future research should explore this issue.

Although the evidence for mental health impacts associated with orphanhood in high-HIV contexts seems clear, very few studies allow comparison of AIDS-orphaned children to other-orphaned children. One of the only large studies that did (Cluver, Fincham, & Seedat, 2009; Cluver et al., 2007; Cluver, Gardner, & Operario, 2008) found that AIDS orphanhood has stronger negative impacts on mental health than orphanhood by other causes (even homicide), as shown in Figure 3.2. However, there is very little longitudinal evidence to allow us to understand how the effects of AIDS orphanhood change over time. In the past two years, a small number of studies have suggested that orphanhood may be associated with an increased likelihood of HIV infection in later life. A recent review

(Cluver & Operario, 2008) found four studies worldwide that reported higher levels of HIV infection among adolescent orphans in Zimbabwe (Birdthistle et al., 2008; Gregson et al., 2005), South Africa (Operario, Pettifor, Cluver, MacPhail, & Rees, 2007) and Russia (Kissin et al., 2007). Further studies reported higher levels of sexual risk behavior (Campbell, Handa, Moroni, Odongo, & Palermo, 2008; Juma, Askew, & Ferguson, 2007; Nyamukapa et al., 2008; Operario et al., 2007; Palermo & Peterman, 2009; Thurman, Brown, Richter, Maharaj, & Magnani, 2006). While there may be varied causes of this higher risk, one study in Zimbabwe does suggest that mental health distress may be contributing to sexual risk behavior among orphans (Nyamukapa et al., 2008).

Children Living with AIDS-Sick and HIV+ Parents or Guardians

Orphanhood by HIV is not a single acute event, rather it is a process preceded by a parent's chronic and debilitating illness (Richter, Foster, & Sherr, 2006). This illness is also often a "family secret"; limiting children's scope to find support outside the family. Furthermore, actually informing children about a parent's HIV status is not simple. Many children report anger, fear and shock when a parent discloses that they have a life-threatening illness. A U.S. study found that children to whom their mothers had disclosed showed more behavioral problems after disclosure (Shaffer, Jones, Kotchick, Forehand, & Family Health Project Research Group, 2001). Despite this, it is generally agreed that disclosure to children is both helpful and necessary for long-term family coping.

Very little is known about the group of children living with HIV+ or AIDS-sick caregivers. In sub-Saharan Africa, studies of children in households with a sick adult do seem to show higher morbidity, malnutrition (Mishra, Arnold, Otieno, Cross, & Hong, 2007), and school absence (Gray et al., 2006), but these studies do not examine mental health. However, there is some evidence that risks to children's emotional well-being may be independently associated with caregiver sickness. For example, in South Africa, the extent of caregiver sickness was shown to mediate levels of mental health problems in uninfected children (Cluver, Gardner et al., 2009). Another small South African study reported higher levels of mental distress among children of parents with full-blown AIDS in comparison with those whose parents did not (Gwandure, 2007). Similarly, studies in the United States have reported that children of HIV-infected parents (particularly adolescents) also experience emotional and behavioral problems (Armistead & Forehand, 1995; Forehand, Armistead, Mose,

Simon, & Clarl, 1998; Forehand et al., 2002; Hudis, 1995; Rotheram-Borus et al., 1999). Understanding the extent to which the mental health problems experienced by AIDS-orphaned children are established during the period of parental sickness is of the utmost importance and is an avenue for future research.

Young Carers

In the West, there is increasing advocacy and evidence to suggest that children who provide care at home for sick parents or siblings are at risk of mental health problems (Becker, 2007; Dearden & Becker, 2000; Levine et al., 2005). These children are often called "young carers" and include children looking after mentally ill, disabled, or substance-using parents. The tasks that these children engage in include household tasks, medical care, and providing emotional support. Due to general limitations in health services, it is likely that many children in sub-Saharan Africa who live with AIDS-unwell caregivers are acting as young carers (see Figure 3.3 for an example); however, there is very little research examining this potentially vulnerable group of children. In the context of the AIDS epidemic, there are no reliable data on the numbers or proportions of children providing such care or on the nature and extent of the tasks that they undertake (e.g., medical, intimate, or emotional care, and care of younger siblings) (Bauman et al., 2006).

One quantitative study (Bauman et al., 2006) compared 50 young carers of AIDS-sick parents in Zimbabwe to 50 young carers in the United States. Results revealed high levels of depression in both groups. Interestingly,

Figure 3.3
Picture and annotation by a young South African girl

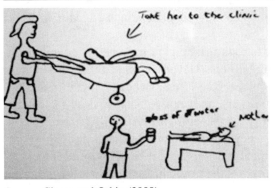

"I take my mother to the clinic in a wheelbarrow. I bring her water when she is in bed" (Girl, 8, urban South Africa).

Source: Cluver and Orkin (2009).

mental health did not seem to be related to extent of caregiving done by children, but future studies with comparison groups of children in healthy homes or homes with other sickness may help to shed further light on this issue. In sub-Saharan Africa, very few studies (all of which are qualitative in nature) have explored children's perceptions of the impact of caregiving (Evans & Becker, 2009; Robson, 2000; Skovdal, Ogutu, Aoro, & Campbell, 2009). In these studies, children have reported both emotional distress and positive experiences and competencies associated with responsibility and contribution to the household. One large-scale, ongoing quantitative study is examining the impacts of being a young carer in the context of HIV/AIDS (Cluver, Kgankga, & Kuo, 2010).

HIV+ Children

Children living in AIDS-affected families may themselves also be infected with HIV. This section will only focus on children who have been infected perinatally (i.e., by an HIV+ parent at birth) as mental health issues may be different for children infected via abuse, drugs, injection drug use, infected blood, and consensual or forced sexual contact.

Before the introduction of pediatric antiretroviral medication, few perinatally infected children survived infancy (Newell et al., 2004). The limited evidence available shows risks of major developmental, motor and emotional delays due to the effect of the virus on the developing brain and nervous system (Richter, Stein, & Cluver, 2009). A recent review of HIV and mental health in sub-Saharan Africa (Jaros, Myer, & Joska, 2009) found nine studies of neurocognitive impacts of parental HIV but very few studies that look at children over two years old or at psychological impacts beyond motor skills and cognitive and neurological abnormalities. Those that did found that HIV+ children scored lower on the personality-social domain of the Denver scale (Boivin et al., 1995) and had less secure attachment to their mothers (Peterson, Drotar, Olness, Guay, & Kiziri Mayengo, 2001).

In the United States, antiretroviral medicine has been provided to infected children since the mid-1990s (Havens et al., 2002). In southern Africa, rollout of ART to infants and children has been far slower, and has been hampered by difficulties such as lack of pediatric dose tablets and complexities in administering suspension formulations. However, with increasing coverage and efficacy of infant and child antiretroviral medicine, it is possible to anticipate that this will be a substantial future demographic group for antiretroviral therapy. This pattern of ART provision in southern Africa, a number of years behind other regions, suggests that we can valuably look to the United States and Europe for indications of potential future challenges.

In the United States (particularly major cities such as New York), ARV provision to infants has resulted in a cohort that has been on anti-retroviral medication since birth and are now moving into adolescence (Bush-Parker, 2000). These adolescents show high levels of mental health problems as they adjust to the reality of a chronic, highly stigmatized, parentally acquired disease (Mellins et al., 2006). In the light of this, there are increasing concerns regarding the negotiation of sexual relationships for this group, including disclosure to sexual partners and safe sex. Clini-cal observation and a small number of studies have noted that the process of adolescent assertion of independence and "acting out" may include rejection of and/or inconsistent use of medication (Mellins, Brackis-Cott, Dolezal, & Abrams, 2004). This may also be because of some of the side effects of ART medicines, such as the developing of fat deposits, make teenagers feel awkward and look different. It is extremely dangerous for children or young people to stop taking ART medication, take it irregu-larly, or miss doses. Not only do they immediately become more likely to get ill from AIDS-related illnesses, but by missing doses they can build up viral resistance, and the HIV virus becomes able to multiply despite the ARV medication.

It is unrealistic to presume that the difficulties for perinatally infected infants, children, and adolescents in southern Africa will be identical to those experienced by perinatally infected children in the United States. However, it may be useful to examine closely the experience of the devel-oped world with this group, to attempt to learn lessons from this work, and put in place interventions based on this research. In particular, it may be important to develop early methods of communication to children regard-ing their HIV status and their antiretroviral use, as a major issue for HIV+ children in both sub-Saharan Africa and elsewhere is that of disclosure. Most children who have been infected with HIV at birth are not told of their HIV status until they are thought to be old enough to understand (and often to keep the family secret). Disclosure to children of their own HIV status often also means disclosure of the parent's HIV status. Research has revealed that disclosure to children of their own HIV status often causes anger toward the parent, resentment and fear, and can disrupt family life for some time. However, children agree that disclosure is important, and many have already guessed by the time they are told of their own HIV status (Armistead et al., 1999; Shaffer et al., 2001).

RISK AND PROTECTIVE FACTORS: DEVELOPING INTERVENTIONS

It is important to develop effective interventions in order to help communities cope with the effects of familial HIV on children's mental health. In order to do this, it is essential to understand the *mechanisms* through which having a caregiver with HIV impacts on child mental health and well-being. What is it about HIV infection, AIDS sickness, and death that render children especially vulnerable? Only a few studies specifically examine potential mechanisms through which parental HIV/AIDS illness influences children's mental health. There is also a lack, as yet, of longitudinal data that would allow stronger inferences to be made about causal relationships between risk and protective factors and child outcomes; having reasonable confidence in these causal paths is vital for program and policy design. While there are many programs and policies that aim to improve mental health for AIDS-affected children, very few of these have been empirically evaluated. In this section we will look at (1) potential mechanisms through which familial HIV may influence child well-being and (2) evidence for what can be effective in improving children's mental health outcomes.

Caregiver Sickness and Effects of HIV

To the best of our knowledge, no known studies have examined the effects of maternal HIV on parenting and childcare; however, two separate bodies of research suggest that HIV/AIDS may compromise parenting ability. Firstly, there is evidence that HIV diagnosis and illness is associated with depression and reduced social support (Stein et al., 2005) and secondly that infants are negatively affected by parental depression and reduced social support (Stein, Ramchanani, & Murray, 2008). Interestingly, one study in South Africa reported that the extent of caregiver illness positively predicted the level of mental health problems in children, but this group of caregivers included both AIDS-sick parents and elderly grandparents (Cluver, Gardner, et al., 2009). Caregiver sickness can limit parental attention, monitoring, and bonding between child and caregiver, thus raising the likelihood of mental health problems and risk behaviors in children.

AIDS-Exacerbated Poverty

As discussed previously, AIDS illness and death have direct and major implications for family poverty. In South Africa, lack of adequate nutrition, school nonattendance (due to financial reasons), and lack of access to social welfare grants were strong mediating factors of mental health problems in AIDS-orphaned children (Cluver & Orkin, 2009). We know far less about the effects of poverty on children living with HIV+ parents or on children who are themselves HIV+, although current research is beginning to address these issues. Children affected by AIDS-exacerbated poverty might be more prone to assume adult responsibilities—both within and outside the home—and experience premature exposure to adult behaviors including sexual risk taking. Indeed, four studies conducted in sub-Saharan Africa have found evidence for earlier sexual debut in orphaned adolescents (e.g., Operario et al., 2007; Thurman et al., 2006).

AIDS-Related Stigma

One of the strongest predictors of mental health problems among AIDS-orphaned children is AIDS-related stigma. A qualitative study in Scotland found that children of HIV+ parents were particularly hurt by people accusing their parents of being promiscuous or prostitutes (Strode & Barrett Grant, 2001). In South Africa, children reporting experience of AIDS-related stigma in the community show far higher levels of depression, peer problems and posttraumatic stress (Cluver et al., 2008). Stigma seems to be directed both at the HIV+ person, and at families of HIV+ people, and is often based on misguided fears of infection through socializing, sharing food or touching a person from an AIDS-affected family (Deacon, 2006; Nyblade, 2006; Strode & Barrett Grant, 2001).[1] We still know very little about how to reduce stigma and discrimination toward the families of HIV+ individuals. Reviews of strategies aiming to reduce stigma for HIV+ individuals suggest potential positive results of legal protection, availability of antiretroviral medication, sensitization and contact with HIV+ people (Brown, Macintyre, & Trujillo, 2003; Klein, Karchner, & O'Connell, 2002); however, to the best of our knowledge no studies have examined the effects of stigma reduction strategies on the *children* of HIV+ parents.

Cumulative Factors

Many theoretical models of child mental health use a "cumulative risk" approach (Rutter, 2000). This suggests that, while children can often cope with a single stressor, multiple stressors can interact to put children at risk of psychological distress. There is little available research to show whether this is true of AIDS-affected children, but a recent study demonstrates interactive and cumulative effects of AIDS-related stigma and undernutrition on orphaned children (Cluver & Orkin, 2009). Those with enough to eat and no stigma had a 19% likelihood of clinical-level disorder, while those experiencing both stigma and hunger had an 83% likelihood (see Figure 3.4). Better understanding of cumulative factors that contribute to mental health problems among AIDS-affected children can guide the specific timing and focus of interventions.

Interventions

There are very few rigorous evaluations of intervention programs designed to improve mental health among AIDS-affected children. In the United States, Rotheram-Borus and her colleagues have reported that a group-based psychological intervention that targets HIV+ parents and their children has long-term positive effects on children's mental health (Rotheram-Borus et al., 2006). Similarly, a recent study (Kumakech, Cantor-Graae, & Maling, 2009) showed positive mental health effects of therapeutic groups for AIDS-orphaned children. While most programs use a counseling or support group–based approach, to the best of our knowledge, there are no studies examining effects of reducing poverty and stigma, and supporting parenting for AIDS-sick parents, on children's

Figure 3.4
Clinical-level disorder among 1,200 children in South Africa

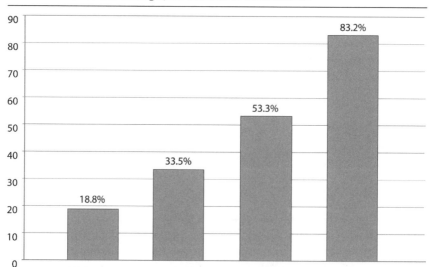

Source: Cluver and Orkin (2009).

mental health and well-being. However, non-HIV studies in other parts of the world suggest that these could have direct benefits on child emotional health (Aber et al., 2007). In other disadvantaged communities, carefully planned short-term psychosocial interventions during pregnancy and the postnatal period can result in long-term mental health benefits to children (Richter et al., 2009). A number of trials in non-HIV contexts have shown that school-based interventions can also be effective at improving social-emotional development in high and low income countries, and have the advantage of being potentially scalable and feasible in some resource-poor settings (Baker-Henningham, Walker, Powell, & Meeks-Gardner, 2009). Similarly, studies of the effects of child-focused cash transfers in other poor communities show long-term educational benefits, although mental health benefits are not tested (Paxson & Schady, 2007). Finally, the provision of antiretroviral medication to HIV+ parents has been shown to have effects on nutrition and growth of their uninfected children (Graff Zivin, Thirumurthy, & Goldstein, 2009), but effects on child mental health have not yet been examined. In the sub-Saharan African context of a generalized HIV epidemic with severe resource constraints, small-scale interventions may not be practical or may not have effects commensurate with the level of need. Policy makers, and increasingly the research community, are accepting that interventions are not sustainable on a large scale unless they are based in existing structures such as NGOs, and make use of existing capacity. However, the vast majority of provision to AIDS-affected children still lacks basic pre- and postmeasurements of outcome, let alone well-controlled evaluations, or evaluation of effects of interventions on key developmental outcomes.

SUMMARY

While there has been a growth in studies from sub-Saharan Africa on the impacts of parental HIV on children, almost all these studies come from a small set of countries—South Africa, Zimbabwe, and Uganda. There are substantial inadequacies in information from elsewhere in the region, as well as in areas of emerging epidemics such as India, China, and Eastern Europe.

From the evidence we do have, it is clear that HIV affects different communities in different ways; however, the impact of parental death by AIDS on children's mental health and well-being appears remarkably consistent across cultures. Children orphaned by AIDS are clearly at increased risk of emotional problems such as depression, anxiety, and post-traumatic stress disorder. However, whether these children are at greater risk than children orphaned by other means is still being investigated, although one large controlled study suggests that this is the case in South Africa (Cluver, Gardner, Operario, 2007). The risk of behavioral problems in AIDS orphans is less clear and based largely on data obtained in the United States. In contrast, very little is known about children living with HIV+ parents or guardians. Many of these children are likely to be "young carers" who are potentially highly vulnerable. This is a group that clearly warrants further investigation. We also know that children who are themselves HIV infected, may experience neurological difficulties, negative social effects (due to stigma associated with the disease), as well as emotional distress (perhaps related to disclosure).

At present the mechanisms through which familial HIV/AIDS impacts on children's mental health are not well understood. Studies suggest AIDS-related stigma, poverty, and caregiver illness may predict mental health outcomes; however further research is clearly needed to document this conclusively. In addition to studying risks, research on protective factors and psychosocial assets can help inform interventions to promote resilience and build on the strengths of children, families, and communities.

Additionally, the vast majority of intervention programs aiming to improve psychological health among AIDS-affected children have not yet been empirically evaluated. This should be a high priority for future research. There are a large number of NGO-led interventions which could valuably be assessed which, if effective, could inform future program design. Despite the extent and duration of the AIDS epidemic, we are still desperately in need of research to guide social policy and programming for children orphaned by AIDS or living with AIDS-sick parents.

NOTE

1. Until recently, there were no validated measures of experience of AIDS-related stigma for uninfected children. A measure has been developed in the United States (Mason, Berger, Ferrans, Sultzman, & Fendrich, 2010) and has been adapted and validated for southern Africa.

REFERENCES

Aber, L., Jones, S., & Raver, C. (2007). Poverty and child development: New perspectives on a defining issue. In L. Aber, S. Bishop-Josef, S. Jones, K. Taaffe McLearn, & D. Phillips (Eds.), *Child development and social policy*. Washington, DC: American Psychological Association.

Anderson, B., & Phillips, H. (2006). *Trends in the percentage of children who are orphaned in South Africa: 1995–2005* (Report No. 03-09-06). Pretoria, South Africa: Statistics SA.

Antinori, A., Arendt, G., Becker, J., Brew, B., Byrd, D., Cherner, M., et al. (2007). Updated research nosology for HIV-associated neurocognitive disorders. *Neurology 69*(18), 1789–1799.

Armistead, L., & Forehand, R. (1995). For whom the bell tolls: Parenting decisions and challenges faced by mothers who are HIV infected. *Clinical Psychology: Science and Practice, 2,* 239–250.

Armistead, L., Summers, P., Forehand, R., Simon Morse, P., Morse, E., & Clark, L. (1999). Understanding of HIV/AIDS among children of HIV-infected mothers: Implications for prevention, disclosure and bereavement. *Children's Health Care, 28*(4), 277–295.

Atwine, B., Cantor-Graae, E., & Bajunirwe, F. (2005). Psychological distress among AIDS orphans in rural Uganda. *Social Science and Medicine, 61*(3), 555–564.

Baker-Henningham, H., Walker, S., Powell, C., & Meeks-Gardner, J. (2009). A pilot study of the Incredible Years Teacher Training Programme and a curriculum unit on social and emotional skills in community preschools in Jamaica. *Child Care Health and Development, 33,* 624–631.

Barnett, T., & Whiteside, A. (2002). *AIDS in the twenty-first century: Disease and globalization.* Basingstoke, UK: Palgrave Macmillan.

Bauman, L., Foster, G., Silver, E. J., Berman, R., Gamble, I., & Muchaneta, L. (2006). Children caring for their ill parents with HIV/AIDS. *Vulnerable Children and Youth Studies, 1*(1), 56–70.

Becker, S. (2007). Global perspectives on children's unpaid caregiving in the family: Research and policy on "young carers" in the UK, Australia, the USA and Sub-Saharan Africa. *Global Social Policy, 7*(1), 23–50.

Bhargava, A. (2005). AIDS epidemic and the psychological well-being and school participation of Ethiopian orphans. *Psychology, Health, and Medicine, 10*(3), 263–275.

Birdthistle, I., Floyd, S., Machingura, A., Mudziwapasi, N., Gregson, S., & Glynn, J. (2008). From affected to infected? Orphanhood and HIV risk among female adolescents in urban Zimbabwe. *AIDS, 22,* 759–766.

Black, D., & Harris-Hendricks, K. (1992). Father kills mother: Post-traumatic stress disorder in the children. *Psychotherapy and Psychosomatics, 57,* 152–157.

Boivin, M., Green, S., Davies, A., Giordani, B., Mokili, J., & Cutting, W. (1995). A preliminary evaluation of the cognitive and motor effects on pediatric HIV infection in Zairian children. *Health Psychology, 14*(1), 13–21.

Booysen, F. (2002). Financial responses of households in the Free State province to HIV/AIDS-related morbidity and mortality. *South African Journal of Economics, 70*(7), 1193–1215.

Brandt, R. (2009). The mental health of people living with HIV/AIDS in Africa: A systematic review. *African Journal of AIDS Research, 8*(2), 123–133.

Bronfenbrenner, U. (1979). *The ecology of human development: Experiments by nature and design.* Cambridge, MA: Harvard University Press.

Brookes, H., Shishana, O., & Richter, L. (2004). *National Household HIV Prevalence and Risk Survey of South African children.* Cape Town: Human Sciences Research Council.

Brown, L., Macintyre, K., & Trujillo, L. (2003). Interventions to reduce HIV/AIDS stigma: What have we learned? *AIDS Education and Prevention, 15*(1), 49–69.

Bush-Parker, T. (2000). Perinatal HIV: Children with HIV grow up. *Focus, 15*(2), 1–4.

Campbell, P., Handa, S., Moroni, M., Odongo, S., & Palermo, T. (2008). *A situation analysis of orphans in 11 eastern and southern African countries.* Nairobi: UNICEF ESARO.

Case, A., & Ardington, C. (2005). *The impact of parental death on school enrolment and achievement: Longitudinal evidence from South Africa* (CSSR Working Paper No. 97). Cape Town: Centre for Social Science Research, University of Cape Town.

Centers for Disease Control and Prevention. (2007). *HIV/AIDS Surveillance Report 2007.* Retrieved from http://www.cdc.gov/hiv/topics/surveillance/resources/reports/2006report/pdf/2006SurveillanceReport.pdf.

Centers for Disease Control and Prevention. (2009). *CDC fact sheet: HIV and AIDS among gay and bisexual men.* Retrieved from http://www.cdc.gov/hiv/resources/factsheets/.

Cluver, L., Fincham, D., & Seedat, S. (2009). Predictors of post-traumatic stress symptomology amongst AIDS-orphaned children. *Journal of Traumatic Stress, 22*(2), 102–112.

Cluver, L., Gardner, F., & Operario, D. (2007). Psychological distress amongst AIDS-orphaned children in urban South Africa. *Journal of Child Psychology and Psychiatry, 48*(8), 755–763.

Cluver, L., Gardner, F., & Operario, D. (2008). Effects of stigma and other community factors on the mental health of AIDS-orphaned children. *Journal of Adolescent Health, 42,* 410–417.

Cluver, L., Gardner, F., & Operario, D. (2009). Caregiving and psychological distress of AIDS-orphaned children. *Vulnerable Children and Youth Studies, 4*(3), 185–199.

Cluver, L., Kgankga, M., & Kuo, C. (2010). *Parenting, disability and HIV/AIDS: Understanding impacts on children in AIDS-affected families.* Paper presented at the Children and HIV: Family Support First—Working Together to Achieve Universal Support and Access to Treatment: IAS Conference, Vienna, Austria.

Cluver, L., & Operario, D. (2008). Review: Intergenerational linkages of AIDS: Vulnerability of orphaned children for HIV infection. *Institute of Development Studies Bulletin, 39*(5), 28–35.

Cluver, L., & Orkin, M. (2009). Cumulative risk and AIDS-orphanhood: Interactions of stigma, bullying, and poverty on child mental health in South Africa. *Social Science and Medicine, 69*(8), 1186–1193.

Deacon, H. (2006). Towards a sustainable theory of health-related stigma: Lessons from the HIV/AIDS literature. *Journal of Community and Applied Social Psychology, 16*(6), 418–425.

Dearden, C., & Becker, S. (2000). *Growing up caring: Vulnerability and transition to adulthood—young carers' experiences.* Leicester, UK: Youth Work Press for the Joseph Rowntree Foundation.

Des Jarlais, D. C., Perlis, T., Arasteh, K., Torian, L. V., Beatrice, S., Milliken, J., et al. (2005). HIV incidence among injection drug users in New York City, 1990 to 2002: Use of serologic test algorithm to assess expansion of HIV prevention services. *American Journal of Public Health, 95*(8), 1439–1444.

Dowdney, L. (2000). Annotation: Childhood bereavement following parental death. *Journal of Child Psychology and Psychiatry, 41*(7), 819–830.

Dowdney, L., Wilson, R., Maughan, B., Allerton, M., Schofield, P., & Skuse, D. (1999). Bereaved children: Psychological disturbance and service provision. *British Medical Journal, 319*, 354–357.

Dunkle, K., Jewkes, R., Brown, H., Gray, G., McIntryre, J., & Harlow, S. (2004). Gender-based violence, relationship power, and risk of HIV infection in women attending antenatal clinics in South Africa. *The Lancet, 363*(9419), 1415–1421.

Evans, J., & Becker, S. (2009). *Children caring for parents with HIV and AIDS: Global issues and policy responses.* Bristol, UK: Policy Press.

Ferreira, M., Keikelame, M., & Mosaval, Y. (2001). *Older women as carers to children and grandchildren affected by AIDS: A study towards supporting the carers.* Cape Town: University of Cape Town, Institute of Ageing in Africa.

Forehand, R., Armistead, L., Mose, E., Simon, P., & Clarl, L. (1998). The Family Health Project: An investigation of children whose mothers are HIV infected. *Journal of Consulting and Clinical Psychology, 66*(3), 513–520.

Forehand, R., Jones, D., Kotchick, B., Armistead, L., Morse, E., Simon Morse, P., et al. (2002). Noninfected children of HIV-infected mothers: A 4-year longitudinal study of child psychosocial adjustment and parenting. *Behavior Therapy, 33*, 579–600.

Forehand, R., Pelton, J., Chance, M., Armistead, L., Morse, E., Morse, P., et al. (1999). Orphans of the AIDS epidemic in the United States: Transition-related characteristics and psychosocial adjustment at 6 months after mother's death. *AIDS Care, 6*, 715–722.

Forrest, G., Plumb, C., Ziebland, S., & Stein, A. (2006). Breast cancer in the family—children's perceptions of their mother's cancer and its initial treatment: Qualitative study. *British Medical Journal, 332*(7548), 998–1003.

Graff Zivin, J., Thirumurthy, H., & Goldstein, M. (2009). AIDS treatment and Intrahousehold resource allocation: Children's nutrition and schooling in Kenya. *Journal of Public Economics, 93*, 1008–1015.

Gray, G. E., Van Niekerk, R., Struthers, H., Violari, A., Martinson, N., McIntyre, J., et al. (2006). The effects of adult morbidity and mortality on household welfare and the well-being of children in Soweto. *Vulnerable Children and Youth Studies, 1*(1), 15–28.

Green, G., & Smith, R. (2004). The psychosocial and health care needs of HIV-positive people in the United Kingdom: A review. *HIV Medicine, 5*(Suppl. 1), 5–46.

Gregson, S., Nyamukapa, C., Garnett, G., Wambe, M., Lewis, J., & Mason, P. (2005). HIV infection and reproductive health in teenage women made vulnerable by AIDS in Zimbabwe. *AIDS Care, 17*(7), 785–794.

Gwandure, C. (2007). Home-based care for parents with AIDS: Impact on children's psychological functioning. *Journal of Child and Adolescent Mental Health, 19*(1), 29–44.

Havens, J., Mellins, C., & Hunter, J. (2002). Psychiatric aspects of HIV/AIDS in childhood and adolescence. In M. Rutter & E. Taylor (Eds.), *Child and adolescent psychiatry: Modern approaches* (4th ed., pp. 828–841). Oxford: Blackwell.

Hudis, J. (1995). Adolescents living in families with AIDS. In S. Geballe, J. Gruendal, & W. Andiman (Eds.), *Forgotten children of the AIDS epidemic* (pp. 83–94). New Haven, CT: Yale University Press.

Hudson, C. (1996). AIDS in rural South Africa: A paradigm for HIV-1 prevention. *International Journal of STD and AIDS, 7*, 236–243.

Hunter, S. (1990). Orphans as a window on the AIDS epidemic in sub-Saharan Africa: Initial results and implications of a study in Uganda. *Social Science and Medicine, 31*(6), 681–690.

Jaros, E., Myer, L., & Joska, J. (2009). *HIV/AIDS and mental health in sub-Saharan Africa: A systematic review* (Unpublished master's of public health thesis). University of Capetown, South Africa.

Juma, M., Askew, I., & Ferguson, A. (2007). *Situation analysis of the sexual and reproductive health and HIV risks and prevention needs of older orphaned and vulnerable children in Nyanza Province, Kenya.* Nairobi: Department of Children's Services, Government of Kenya.

Kissin, D., Zapata, L., Yorick, R., Vinogradova, E., Volkova, G., Cherkassova, E., et al. (2007). HIV seroprevalence in street youth, St. Petersburg, Russia. *AIDS, 21*, 2333–2340.

Klein, S., Karchner, W., & O'Connell, D. (2002). Interventions to prevent HIV-related stigma and discrimination: Findings and recommendations for public health practice. *Journal of Public Health Management and Practice, 8*(6), 44–53.

Kumakech, E., Cantor-Graae, E., & Maling, S. (2009). Peer-group support intervention improves the psychosocial well-being of AIDS orphans: Cluster randomized trial. *Social Science and Medicine, 68*(6), 1038–1043.

Kuo, C., & Operario, D. (2009a). Caring for AIDS-orphaned children: A systematic review of studies on caregivers. *Vulnerable Children and Youth Studies, 4*(1), 1–12.

Kuo, C., & Operario, D. (2011). Health of adults caring for orphaned children in an HIV-endemic community in South Africa. *AID Care,* DOI: 10.1080/09540121.2011.554527.

Levine, C., Gibson Hunt, G., Halper, D., Hart, A. Y., Lautz, J., & Gould, D. (2005). Young adult caregivers: A first look at an unstudied population. *American Journal of Public Health, 95*(11), 2071–2075.

Luthar, S., Cicchetti, D., & Becker, B. (2000). The construct of resilience: A critical evaluation and guidelines for future work. *Child Development, 71*(3), 543–562.

Makame, V., Ani, C., & McGregor, S. (2002). Psychological well-being of orphans in Dar El-Salaam, Tanzania. *Acta Paediatrica, 91*, 459–465.

Mason, S., Berger, B., Ferrans, C. E., Sultzman, V., & Fendrich, M. (2010). Developing a measure of stigma by association with African American adolescents whose mothers have HIV. *Research on Social Work Practice, 20*(1), 65–73.

Mellins, C., Brackis-Cott, E., Abrams, E., & Dolezal, C. (2006). Rates of psychiatric disorder in perinatally HIV-infected youth. *Pediatric Infectious Disease Journal, 25*, 432–437.

Mellins, C., Brackis-Cott, E., Dolezal, C., & Abrams, E. (2004). The role of psychosocial and family factors in adherence to antiretroviral treatment in Human Immunodeficiency Virus–infected children. *Pediatric Infectious Disease Journal, 23*, 1035–1041.

Mellins, C. A., Elkington, K. S., Bauermeister, J. A., Brackis-Cott, E., Dolezal, C., McKay, M., et al. (2009). Sexual and drug use behavior in perinatally HIV-infected youth: Mental health and family influences. *Journal of the American Academy of Child and Adolescent Psychiatry, 48*(8), 810–819.

Mishra, V., Arnold, F., Otieno, F., Cross, A., & Hong, R. (2007). Education and nutritional status of orphans and children of HIV-infected parents in Kenya. *AIDS Education and Prevention, 19*(5), 383–395.

Newell, M.-L., Coovadia, H., Cortina-Borja, M., Rollins, N., Gaillard, P., & Dabis, F. (2004). Mortality of infected and uninfected infants born to HIV-infected mothers in Africa: A pooled analysis. *The Lancet, 3641*, 1236–1243.

Nyamukapa, C., Gregson, S., Lopman, B., Saito, S., Watts, H., Monasch, R., et al. (2008). HIV-associated orphanhood and children's psychosocial distress: Theoretical framework tested with data from Zimbabwe. *American Journal of Public Health, 98*(1), 133–141.

Nyblade, N. (2006). Measuring HIV stigma: Existing knowledge and gaps. *Psychology, Health, and Medicine, 11*(3), 335–345.

Operario, D., Pettifor, A., Cluver, L., MacPhail, C., & Rees, H. (2007). Prevalence of parental death among young people in South Africa and risk for HIV infection. *Journal of Acquired Immune Deficiency Syndromes, 44*, 93–98.

Palermo, T., & Peterman, A. (2009). Are female orphans at risk for early marriage, early sexual debut, and teen pregnancy? Evidence from sub-Saharan Africa. *Studies in Family Planning, 40*, 101–112.

Paxson, C., & Schady, N. (2007). *Does money matter? The effects of cash transfers on child health and development in rural Ecuador* (World Bank Policy Research Working Paper No. 1–43). Washington, DC: World Bank.

Peterson, N., Drotar, D., Olness, K., Guay, L., & Kiziri Mayengo, R. (2001). The relationship of maternal and child HIV infection to security of attachment among Ugandan infants. *Child Psychiatry and Human Development, 32*(1), 3–17.

Richter, L., Foster, G., & Sherr, L. (2006). *Where the heart is: Meeting the psychosocial needs of young children in the context of HIV/AIDS.* Toronto, ON, Canada: Bernard Van Leer Foundation.

Richter, L., Stein, A., & Cluver, L. (2009). Infants and young children affected by AIDS. In P. Rohleder, L. Swartz, S. Kalichman, & L. Simbayi (Eds.), *HIV/ AIDS in South Africa 25 years on: Psychosocial perspectives* (pp. 69–88). New York: Springer.

Robson, E. (2000). Invisible carers: Young people in Zimbabwe's home-based healthcare. *Area, 32*(1), 59–69.

Rochat, T., Richter, L., Doll, H., Buthelezi, N., Tomkins, A., & Stein, A. (2006). Depression among pregnant rural South African women undergoing HIV testing. *Journal of the American Medical Association, 295*(12), 1376–1378.

Rotheram-Borus, M. J., Lee, M., Lin, Y. Y., & Lester, P. (2004). Six-year intervention outcomes for adolescent children of parents with the Human Immunodeficiency Virus. *Archives of Pediatric and Adolescent Medicine, 158*, 742–748.

Rotheram-Borus, M., Lester, P., Song, J., Lin, Y., Leonard, N., Beckwith, L., et al. (2006). Intergenerational benefits of family-based HIV interventions. *Journal of Consulting and Clinical Psychology, 74*, 622–627.

Rotheram-Borus, M. J., Lightfoot, M., & Shen, H. (1999). Levels of emotional distress among parents living with AIDS and their adolescent children. *AIDS and Behaviour, 03*(4), 367–372.

Rutter, M. (2000). Psychosocial influences: Critiques, findings, and research needs. *Development and Psychopathology, 12*, 375–405.

Rutter, M. (2006). Implications of resilience concepts for scientific understanding. *Annals of the New York Academy of Sciences, 1094*, 1–12.

Shaffer, A., Jones, D., Kotchick, B., Forehand, R., & Family Health Project Research Group. (2001). Telling the children: Disclosure of maternal HIV infection and its effects on child psychosocial adjustment. *Journal of Child and Family Studies, 10*(3), 301–313.

Simoni, J. M., Davis, M. L., Drossman, J. A., & Weinberg, B. A. (2000). Mothers with HIV/AIDS and their children: Disclosure and guardianship issues. *Women and Health, 31*(1), 39–54.

Skovdal, M., Ogutu, V. O., Aoro, C., & Campbell, C. (2009). Young carers as social actors: Coping strategies of children caring for ailing or ageing guardians in western Kenya. *Social Science and Medicine, 69*(4), 587–595.

Springer, S. A., & Altice, F. L. (2005). Managing HIV/AIDS in correctional settings. *Current HIV/AIDS Reports, 2*(4), 165–170.

Stein, A., Krebs, G., Richter, L., Tomkins, A., Rochat, T., & Bennish, M. (2005). Babies of a pandemic: Infant development and HIV. *Archives of the Diseases of Childhood, 90*, 116–118.

Stein, A., Ramchandani, P., & Murray, L. (2008). Impact of parental psychiatric disorder or physical illness. In M. Rutter, D. Bishop, D. Pine, S. Scott, J. Stevenson, E. Taylor, et al. (Eds.), *Rutter's child and adolescent psychiatry* (pp. 407–420). Malden, MA: Blackwell.

Strode, A., & Barrett Grant, K. (2001). *The role of stigma and discrimination in increasing the vulnerability of children and youth infected with and affected by HIV/AIDS.* London: Save the Children.

Thurman, T., Brown, L., Richter, L., Maharaj, P., & Magnani, R. (2006). Sexual risk behavior among South African adolescents: Is orphan status a factor? *AIDS and Behavior, 10*(6), 627–635.

UNAIDS. (2008). *Report on the global AIDS epidemic.* Geneva, Switzerland: Author.

Zhao, G., Li, X., Fang, X., Zhao, J., Yang, H., & Stanton, B. (2007). Care arrangement, grief, and psychological problems among children orphaned by AIDS in China. *AIDS Care, 19*(9), 1075–1082.

Chapter 4

POSTNATAL DEPRESSION AND ITS EFFECTS ON CHILD DEVELOPMENT: A DEVELOPING WORLD PERSPECTIVE

Christine E. Parsons, Katherine S. Young,
Peter J. Cooper, and Alan Stein

Depression is the most frequently occurring psychiatric condition among women of childbearing age, with more than 8% being affected at any given time (Weissman et al., 1988). Depression occurring among women specifically in the postnatal period has been the focus of a great deal of research in the developed world for a number of reasons. Postnatal depression is common, with prevalence rates estimated at around 10%–13% in developed countries (O'Hara & Swain, 1996). There is strong evidence from high-income countries to show that postnatal depression raises the risk of adverse outcomes for the mother and her partner, both in terms of the quality of their relationship and a raised risk for partner mental health problems (Boath, Pryce, & Cox, 1998); and family disturbances (Lovestone & Kumar, 1993). Postnatal depression is also associated with impairments in mother–infant interactions, as well as longer-term disruption of emotional and cognitive development of the infant (Murray, Halligan, & Cooper, 2009). An important finding from research in developed countries is that socioeconomic status is a key moderator of the effects of postnatal depression on parenting difficulties and subsequent child development. Thus, in poor economic environments, especially in the context of low levels of social support, parenting difficulties are more likely and the risk of negative child outcomes is raised (e.g., Stein et al., 2008). Until relatively recently, little research has been conducted on postnatal depression in developing and low- and middle-income contexts. The prevalence of socioeconomic adversity in these contexts is high, not only raising the risks for negative effects on children, but also raising the risks for maternal depression itself.

A scientific consensus is emerging that the origins of adult disease are frequently found among developmental and biological disturbances that occur in the early years of life (Shonkoff, Boyce, & McEwen, 2009). The extent to which early experiences are considered formative has been further underlined by the Marmot review (Marmot, 2010) which concludes that giving each child the best start in life is the highest priority for reducing health inequality. Thus, the rearing environment of young children has the potential to have effects on later health and development. In this chapter, we first review the prevalence rates of postnatal depression in developing countries. We then consider what is known about the impact of postnatal depression on children in developing contexts across the domains of physical and psychological development. We consider how the presence of HIV may impact on child development, indirectly by compromising maternal mental health, as well as through direct pathways. Finally, we review the small number of intervention studies conducted in this field. We conclude by considering priorities and strategies for intervention.

PREVALENCE

Although almost 90% of the world's children live in developing countries, far less is known about prevalence rates of postnatal depression (PND) in these countries in comparison to developed countries. However, existing evidence suggests that PND is common and is a substantial risk to child development (Walker et al., 2007). Epidemiological studies have found high rates of depression in developing countries, particularly among women facing socioeconomic difficulties (e.g., Husain, Creed, & Tomenson, 2000). Reliable estimates of the prevalence of postnatal depression in developing contexts are essential to the development of national and international health policies for intervention.

Studies on prevalence rates of depression specifically in the postnatal period in developing countries have found depression rates comparable to, if not significantly higher, than those in high income countries (see Figure 4.1). Different measures have been used to assess depressive disorder. As in the developed world, assessments using diagnostic clinical interviews provide lower estimates than those using screening questionnaires. Figure 4.2 provides a comparison (where available) between such interview and questionnaire measures across developing world countries. The majority of work to date has focused on prevalence rates in Asian

Figure 4.1
Mean prevalence of postnatal depression in developing countries

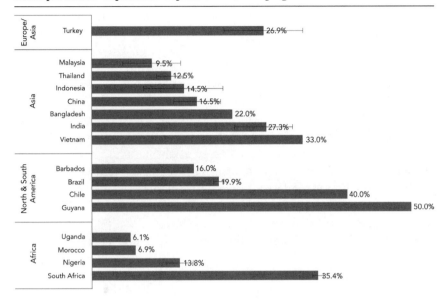

Figure 4.2
Mean prevalence of postnatal depression, comparing rates found using clinical interviews and self-report questionnaires

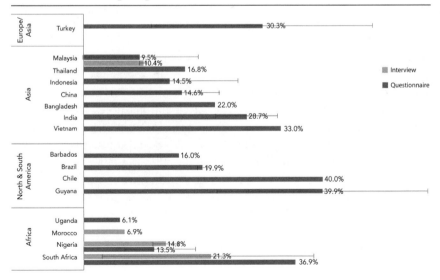

countries, with wide ranges in prevalence reported both within and between countries. In South Asia, estimates of prevalence in India have ranged between 19.8% and 35.5% (e.g., Chandran, Tharyan, Muliyil, & Abraham, 2002); in Pakistan between 28% and 36% (e.g., Husain et al., 2006); in Nepal between 4.9% and 12% (e.g., Ho-Yen, Bondevik, Eberhard-Gran, & Bjorvatn, 2006); and in Bangladesh the rate was estimated at 22% (Gausia, Fisher, Ali, & Oosthuizen, 2009). Similar estimates have been found in Southeast Asia, with prevalence in Vietnam reported at 33% (Fisher, Morrow, Ngoc, & Anh, 2004), in Malaysia between 3.9% and 28.1% (e.g., Mahmud, Shariff, & Yaacob, 2002), in Thailand between 10% and 16.8% (e.g., Liabsuetrakul, Vittayanont, & Pitanupong, 2007), and in Indonesia between 6.6% and 22.4% (e.g., Andajani-Sutjahjo, Manderson, & Astbury, 2007). In the rest of Asia, prevalence in China has been estimated between 7.2% and 25% (e.g., Wang, Jiang, Jan, & Chen, 2003), in Mongolia at 9.1% (Pollock, Manaseki-Holland, & Patel, 2009), and in Lebanon at 21% (Chaaya et al., 2002).

In Africa, a wide range of prevalence ranges have also been reported, with no clear differences between northern and sub-Saharan African countries. In the north, prevalence of postnatal depression in Burkina Faso was estimated at 44% (Baggaley et al., 2007), between 5.6% and 20.1% in Morocco (Agoub, Moussaoui, & Battas, 2005), and between 3.2% and 6.9% in The Gambia (Coleman, Morison, Paine, Powell, & Walraven, 2006). In sub-Saharan regions, prevalence in Ethiopia has been estimated between 13% and 37.1% (e.g., Tesfaye, Hanlon, Wondimagegn, & Alem, 2010), in South Africa between 7.8% and 36.9% (Lawrie, Hofmeyr, De Jager, & Berk, 1998), in Nigeria between 3.7% and 23% (e.g., Owoeye, Aina, & Morakinyo, 2006), between 6.1% and 16% in Uganda (e.g., Nakku, Nakasi, & Mirembe, 2006), at 16% in Zimbabwe (Nhiwatiwa, Patel, & Acuda, 1998), and at 13.9% in Malawi (Stewart et al., 2010).

Prevalence studies both in South America and in Turkey have reported even wider estimate ranges within countries. In Turkey, estimates range from 14% to 50.7% (e.g., Kirpinar, Gozum, & Pasinliolu, 2010); in Chile, from 10.2% to 50% (e.g., Florenzano et al., 2002), in Brazil from 11.4% to 56% (e.g., Surkan, Kawachi, Ryan et al., 2008), and in Guyana from 24.6% to 57% (Affonso, De, Horowitz, & Mayberry, 2000). In Central America, estimates for Costa Rican women have been between 34% and 46% (Wolf, De Andraca, & Lozoff, 2002), and for Barbadian women, 16% (Galler, Harrison, Biggs, Ramsey, & Forde, 1999).

As mentioned earlier, at least part of the variation in prevalence estimates within and across countries may be related to the different screening tools, postnatal stage, and cutoff scores used in these studies. The Edinburgh Postnatal Depression Scale (EPDS) is the most extensively used measure for PND across a wide variety of countries and languages, but other studies have employed structured psychiatric interviews (e.g., Structured Clinical Interview for DSM-IV; SCID), or a range of self-report scales including the Beck Depression Inventory (BDI), revised Clinical Interview Schedule (CIS-R), the WHO self-reporting questionnaire (SRQ), the Centre for Epidemiological Studies depression scale (CES-D), the Mini International Neuropsychiatric Interview (MINI), the Hamilton Depression Rating Scale (HDRS), Zung's self-rating depression scale, and the Kessler scales. These different scales appear to result in quite different estimates, even for the same women at the same time point. For instance, one study in India reported a prevalence of 24.5% using the BDI and 32.4% using the EPDS (Affonso et al., 2000). Similarly, variation of 29.1% in prevalence rates has also been reported when using the DSM-IV criteria compared with the EPDS in a sample in South Africa (Lawrie et al., 1998). The most widely used and stringent cutoff point for the EPDS is above 12. At this cutoff, studies have still reported high prevalence rates (e.g., 50% in Turkey; Alkar & Gencoz, 2005). Other studies have used lower cutoff points, such as scores of greater than 10 and have reported lower prevalence rates (e.g., 22% in Bangladesh; Gausia et al., 2009). There is a clear need for a consensus on best practice cutoff scores and scales if reliable estimates of prevalence are to be obtained.

RISK FACTORS FOR POSTNATAL DEPRESSION

Four systematic reviews have identified the following risk factors for postnatal depression in developed countries: history of any psychopathology (including history of previous PND), a lack of social support, poor marital or partner relationship, and recent negative life events (Beck, 1996; O'Hara & Swain, 1996; Robertson, Grace, Wallington, & Stewart, 2004; Wilson et al., 1996). There is also a raised risk of PND among immigrant populations (Glasser et al., 1998).

While poverty and economic adversity are associated with maternal PND in both developed and developing countries, developing countries are characterized by higher rates of poverty and economic stress than elsewhere. The relatively high prevalence of maternal PND in developing countries may be a result of women's exposure to such risk factors for depression (Broadhead & Abas, 1998) as socioeconomic hardship, and especially in sub-Saharan Africa, the high prevalence of HIV/AIDS (Stein et al., 2005). Furthermore, gender inequalities may be relevant in some areas. For example, research from India has found that disappoint-ment with the birth of a female child is associated with the development of postnatal depression (Chandran, Tharyan, Muliyil, & Abraham, 2002). High rates of postnatal depression in developing countries may also reflect the lack of protective factors that can buffer against the onset of depression. For example, while better educated women are less likely to become depressed than poorly educated women (e.g., Husain et al., 2000), gender inequalities in secondary education are typical in many developing countries.

IMPACT OF POSTNATAL DEPRESSION ON CHILD DEVELOPMENT

In developing countries, carers, particularly the mother, play a critical role in child survival and development. The environment in which moth-ers provide caregiving is typically more adverse than in developed coun-tries, with mothers daily facing great physical burdens. Overcrowding, a lack of running water or electricity and poor sanitation are common. In these circumstances, in addition to initiating and maintaining exclusive breast-feeding until six months, mothers have to manage weaning, hy-giene, water sanitation, and ensuring the child is immunized. If the child becomes unwell, the mother needs to recognize the illness, provide care, obtain external help, and carry out treatment. Clearly, the mother's mental health may play an important role in how well she is able to perform these caregiving behaviors. For example, depression is typically characterized by poor concentration, lethargy, sleep disturbance and low mood, all of which could interfere with a mother's capacity to carry out these tasks.

Until recently, most research on the impact of postnatal depression on child development has derived from populations in developed countries. In this section, we examine whether postnatal depression is associated with disturbances in child health and development in developing world contexts. In developed countries, there has been considerable research on the impact of maternal depression on infant psychological rather than physical development, whereas the reverse is true for developing coun-tries, because physical development is such a major concern.

Infant Physical Health

The best global indicator of a child's well-being is growth, because infections, a lack of food or unsatisfactory feeding practices, or more frequently a combination of these, are principal factors affecting physical growth and cognitive development. A child's body responds to poor nutrition in a number of ways that can be measured using growth indices. Wasting is a short-term response to inadequate nutritional intake and is measured by weight relative to length/height. Stunting is a longer-term response that reflects a deceleration or cessation of growth measured by length/height relative to age. Wasting and stunting therefore discriminate between different processes. Wasting is considered to be the index of choice for severely malnourished children who may be at raised risk of death. Stunting is thought to best reflect the long-term cumulative effects resulting from inadequate diet and/or recurrent illness. A third widely used growth index, weight for age, can reflect either stunting and/or wasting, and therefore does not discriminate between short and longer-term forms of poor nutrition. There is strong evidence that poor growth is associated with impaired cognitive development and deficits in school performance and intellectual achievement (e.g., Grantham-McGregor et al., 2007). Growth impairment in early childhood is also associated with significant functional impairment in adult life (World Health Organization, 1995).

Poor child growth is a major public health problem in developing countries. It has been estimated that more than 220 million children aged less than five years in developing countries have substantially impaired growth (UNICEF, 1998). Recent estimates suggest that stunting, wasting and intrauterine growth restriction are the cause of 2.2 million deaths and 21% of disability-adjusted life years lost among children less than five years old (Black et al., 2008), per annum. Physical development of infants is a particular problem in Asia. In what is referred to as the "Asian enigma," the nutritional status of children in South Asia has been found to be poorer than those of children in Africa, despite comparable economic conditions (Bamalingaswami, Jonsson, & Rohde, 1996). Determinants of the disproportionately higher rates of child undernutrition in this largely food-sufficient area are not well understood. Evidence appears to indicate that as the amount of food available per person increases, its power to reduce child malnutrition weakens (Smith & Haddad, 2000). Consequently, attention has gradually been turning to factors other than nutritional intake, such as maternal behavior and health and sociocultural practices, which may influence child health and development.

A number of recent studies have examined whether maternal depressive symptoms are associated with child nutritional outcomes as indexed by inadequate growth. Overall, findings from these studies have been mixed, with strong associations reported in some regions but not others. Three published studies to date have examined the predictive relationship between maternal mental health problems during pregnancy and child physical outcomes, all based in South Asia. One study of mothers in rural Pakistan found that depressive symptoms during pregnancy were predictive of low birth weight status (Rahman, Bunn, Lovel, & Creed, 2007a). A second study in Pakistan found that prenatal depression in mothers predicted poorer growth outcomes in infants at 2, 6, and 12 months with poorest outcomes for those infants of mothers with persistent depression (Rahman, Iqbal, Bunn, Lovel, & Harrington, 2004). In this study, postnatal depression was also found to have an independent effect on growth outcomes. A third study in India found an association between more broadly defined maternal psychological morbidity and low birth weight (Patel & Prince, 2006). It is interesting that evidence from developed countries for an effect of depressive symptoms during pregnancy on birth weight has been conflicting (e.g., Evans, Heron, Patel, & Wiles, 2007; Field et al., 2004). However, if such an association does exist in developing countries, these infants may be especially vulnerable because low birth weight is itself a risk factor for adverse outcomes; furthermore prenatal maternal depression increases the risk for postpartum depression (Dennis, Janssen, & Singer, 2004), which itself is associated with compromised child development.

Several recent studies from South Asia have reported an association between maternal postnatal depression and concurrent measures of child growth. In a cohort study in Goa, India, postnatal depression between six and eight weeks was an independent predictor of concurrent low weight and length for age (Patel, DeSouza, & Rodrigues, 2003). A study in rural India produced similar findings: infants between 6 and 12 months who were underweight or stunted were more likely to have a mother with depression than infants with normal weight (Anoop, Saravanan, Joseph, Cherian, & Jacob, 2004). In Bangladesh, infants of mothers with high levels of depressive symptoms were more likely to be stunted at 6 and 12 months of age (Black, Baqui, Zaman, Arifeen, & Black, 2009). In Pakistan, one study reported that underweight nine-month-old infants were significantly more likely to have a mother with high levels of distress (defined by the WHO SRQ) than infants of normal weight (Rahman, Lovel, Bunn, Iqbal, & Harrington, 2004). A cross-sectional study in both India and Vietnam found that maternal common mental disorder, as measured by the SRQ, was associated with greater likelihood of stunting and underweight status in infants aged between 6 and 18 months (Harpham, Huttly, De Silva, & Abramsky, 2005).

The association between maternal depressive symptoms and poor infant physical growth has been reported in some countries beyond South Asia but not others. In Jamaica, mothers of infants aged between 9 and

30 months with impaired physical growth (stunting, wasting and under-weight status) had more depressive symptoms than mothers of healthy infants (Baker-Henningham, Powell, Walker, & Grantham-McGregor, 2003). However, when socioeconomic status was taken into account, there was no independent relationship between psychosocial function of the mother and the infant's growth status. In one of the earliest studies of its kind conducted in Brazil, the mothers of underweight infants aged less than two years were more likely to have a mental disturbance than mothers of healthy children (De Miranda et al., 1996). More recent studies of Brazilian mother–infant dyads also found an association between mater-nal depressive symptoms and child growth measures, but the pattern of the relationship was somewhat different; maternal depressive symptoms were associated with stunting in infants aged between 6 and 24 months, but overweight rather than underweight status (Surkan, Kawachi, & Peterson, 2008). A study in Peru found no association between maternal common mental disorder and stunting or weight for age (Harpham et al., 2005).

Findings from sub-Saharan Africa have differed from country to country, with some studies reporting an association and others not. In a longitudinal study in Nigeria, infants of mothers with depression at 6 weeks after birth had significantly poorer growth compared with in-fants of healthy mothers, as measured by weight for age and stunting, at 3 and 6 months, but not at 6 weeks and 9 months (Adewuya, Ola, Aloba, Mapayi, & Okeniyi, 2008). In Malawi, infants of mothers with common mental disorder were more likely to be stunted, but not underweight, than infants with healthy mothers at 9 months of age (Stewart et al., 2008). One study in South Africa found no clear relationship between maternal depressive symptoms and infant stunting or weight for age (Tomlinson, Cooper, Stein, Swartz, & Molteno, 2006). Two very recent studies have examined this issue. A study from Ethiopia found no association between maternal common mental disorder and infant underweight status or infant stunting (Medhin et al., 2010). On the other hand, the birth to 20 longitu-dinal study in Soweto-Johannesburg in South Africa found that postnatal depression was associated with stunting at two years of age, and that stunting mediated the negative effect of postnatal depression on behavior problems (Avan, Ramchandani, Richter, Norris, & Stein, 2010).

It is unclear why maternal depression appears to be related to infant growth in some countries but not others. As indicated earlier, the most robust evidence base for an association between depressive symptoms and impaired growth comes from South Asia. Across countries and cultures, there are considerably different psychosocial experiences associated with the birth of a child, such as in the rates of lone motherhood, the nature of marriage, family and kinship, and variations in the support new mothers receive. It may be that socioeconomic and sociocultural factors interact in determining the effect of maternal mental health on child nutrition. It has been argued that South Asian women have a poorer social status and are less empowered than women elsewhere (Harpham et al., 2005). In such a context, a mother with depression may find it more difficult to secure appropriate nutrition for her infant. In South Asia, infant gender (having a girl) has been shown to be a powerful determinant of maternal mental health difficulties (Patel et al., 2003), which does not appear to be the case in Africa. Other possible reasons include different breast-feeding practices and maternal nutrition, or other social and genetic factors. Further studies are necessary to determine whether antenatal depression has an impact upon birth weight in sub-Saharan Africa and other developing countries and whether this has an impact upon subsequent measures of infant growth. There are several possible mechanisms through which maternal depressive symptoms could be linked to impaired fetal and infant growth including, maternal undernutrition and poor self-care (Rahman, Harrington, & Bunn, 2002), disruption to mother–infant interactions (Cooper et al., 1999), increased rates of infant diarrhea (Rahman, Bunn, Lovel, & Creed, 2007b), and early termination of breast-feeding (Henderson, Evans, Straton, Priest, & Hagan, 2003).

Breast-Feeding

The Global Strategy on Infant and Young Child Feeding recommends, as a critical public health measure, that all infants are breast-fed exclusively up until 6 months of age and that breast-feeding continues with the introduction of appropriate foods up to two years and beyond (World Health Organization, 2003). This recommendation is especially important for developing contexts where the protective effects of breast-feeding are more evident than in developed countries (Cattaneo & Quintero-Romero, 2006). In developed countries, there is strong evidence linking postnatal depression with premature cessation of breast-feeding or suboptimal breast-feeding practices (e.g., Cooper, Murray, & Stein, 1993). Consistent with this, depressive symptoms have been associated with premature cessation of breast-feeding across a number of studies in developing countries. Mothers with depressive symptoms in the first four to six weeks postpartum were likely to stop breast-feeding earlier than nondepressed mothers, both in Nigeria (Adewuya et al., 2008) and in Brazil (Falceto, Giugliani, & Fernandes, 2004). Mood at seven weeks predicted Barbadian mothers' current and future preference for breast-feeding, as well as actual feeding behavior at six months (Galler, Harrison, Ramsey, Chawla, & Taylor, 2006). In Pakistan, the prevalence of depression was higher in a group of mothers who had stopped breast-feeding early than in a group of mothers who continued to breast-feed (Taj & Sikander, 2003). However, two studies have found similar rates of breast-feeding before four months in mothers with and without depression in Brazil (Falccto et al., 2004) and Turkey (Kara, Ünalan, Çifçili, Cebeci, & Sarper, 2008), suggesting that depressive symptoms do not necessarily disrupt breast-feeding. Again, the reasons for the association between maternal depression and breast-feeding duration are unclear, but are likely to be multifactorial.

Diarrhea

Diarrhea is another major public health concern in developing countries. Annually, it kills in the region of 2.2 million people, the majority of whom are infants or young children (World Health Organization, 2000). Preventing diarrhea in infants requires the caregiver, typically the mother, to take sanitation measures and be alert and responsive in the challenging environment of a poor community. Two studies have reported an association between maternal depressive symptoms and infant diarrheal episodes. Infants of depressed mothers had significantly higher rates of diarrhea per year than those of healthy mothers in Pakistan (Rahman et al., 2007b) and in Nigeria, where the infants also had higher rates of other childhood illnesses (Adewuya et al., 2008). However, the link between preventable illnesses such as diarrhea and maternal depressive symptoms requires further investigation. In the regions where this effect has been found, other studies have reported an effect of maternal depressive symptoms on infant physical growth, an effect not found elsewhere (e.g., Tomlinson et al., 2006). Again, there may be sociocultural or environmental factors specific to these regions, or an interaction of these factors that may account for the association.

Cognitive and Emotional Development

Findings from a diverse range of studies in developed countries suggest that postnatal depression, especially if chronic, poses a risk for long-term poor cognitive functioning in the child, particularly in the context of wider socioeconomic difficulties (Murray et al., 2009). While the vast majority of work on the impact of postnatal depression on infant cognitive development has been conducted in high-income settings, there is emerging evidence for an effect in at least some developing countries. In

India, Patel et al. (2003) found that the six-month-old infants of mothers who had postnatal depression at six weeks had significantly lower mental, but not motor, quotient scores, than infants of nondepressed mothers. A study of mothers in Barbados similarly found that postnatal depression at seven weeks predicted lower infant social and cognitive performance at 6 months (Galler, Harrison, Ramsey, Forde, & Butler, 2000). Finally, in Ethiopia, maternal symptoms of mental disorders were negatively associated with their children's scores on personal–social, fine motor, gross motor, and overall development between 3 and 24 months, but not their language scores (Hadley, Tegegn, Tessema, Asefa, & Galea, 2008). The limited number of studies in developing contexts precludes conclusions about the impact of postnatal depression on cognitive development, but given that socioeconomic hardship appears to moderate the impact of maternal depression on infant cognitive development, further studies in this area are clearly warranted.

The capacity of parents to provide the kind of care that promotes secure infant attachment and good psychological developmental in childhood can be compromised in adverse conditions such as poverty, especially in the context of maternal postnatal depression (e.g., Atkinson et al., 2000). This is of particular concern for populations in developing countries. Nonetheless, few studies have examined the emotional and behavioral development of children in the context of postnatal depression in developing countries. One study in South Africa found marked impairments in interactions between dyads where the mother had depression compared with healthy mothers (Cooper et al., 1999). A follow-up study found that these early parenting difficulties were associated with subsequent insecure infant attachment (Tomlinson, Cooper, & Murray, 2005).

HIV, MATERNAL DEPRESSION, AND INFANT OUTCOMES

Although it is increasingly recognized that Asia and parts of Eastern Europe are facing a major HIV problem, the HIV pandemic has been particularly devastating in sub-Saharan Africa where two thirds of the infected people live, and where widespread poverty and poor nutrition already undermine children's health and well-being. Half of the new infections in 2005 occurred in the 15–24 age group, the next generation of parents. In some parts of sub-Saharan Africa up to 50% of women attending antenatal clinics are HIV positive. There is now a body of evidence that indicates that even uninfected children of HIV positive mothers are at increased risk in terms of development (Stein et al., 2005). There is concern that receiving a diagnosis of HIV will impact on the mother's caregiving capacity and that one of the ways that this occurs is because of the effect on her mental state. Thus, being diagnosed with HIV during pregnancy, when most African women learn of their diagnosis, often leads to depression and even suicidal feelings (Rochat et al., 2006). While preparing to bring a new life into the world, the mother is, at the same time, confronted with the prospect of a chronic and potentially fatal illness. Questions hang over the fidelity of her relationships and her future fertility. In addition, the high levels of stigma associated with HIV often disrupt her social and material support networks (e.g., Kwalombota, 2002). The combination of being diagnosed with HIV and being depressed is likely to put particular pressure on a new mother and her parenting and may well have cumulative negative effects on mother–child interaction and the child's development (Stein et al., 2005). While some studies have shown that HIV infection is associated with disturbances in mother–infant interactions (e.g., Kotchick et al., 1997), it is not clear whether this is related to the impact of maternal psychosocial functioning or other factors.

Mediating Mechanisms

There are a number of potential environmental mechanisms through which postnatal depression can adversely affect child outcome. Research primarily from developed countries has shown that depression compromises the quality of the mother's caregiving, and suggests that disturbances in parenting are key mechanisms by which maternal depression affects child development (Murray et al., 2009). There are several related, partially overlapping, dimensions of parenting that have been identified as significant: notably, the missing of infant cues, lack of contingent responsiveness, intrusiveness, and poor facilitation, as well as low parental mood itself (e.g., Stein et al., 1991). Some evidence exists to suggest that in the developing world also, major depression in the postnatal period can have a negative impact upon mother–infant interactions (Cooper et al., 1999), which in turn are related to negative outcomes in infant attachment security (Tomlinson et al., 2005), poor hygiene, gastrointestinal infections and diarrhea. Notably, infants of depressed mothers were less likely to be fully immunized at 12 months compared with infants of nondepressed mothers in Pakistan, possibly indicating a lack of appropriate health-seeking behavior in depressed mothers (Rahman, Iqbal et al., 2004).

Interventions

The question that most urgently needs to be addressed is what can be done to help women and their children, and in particular, what intervention strategies are necessary to minimize the impact of maternal depression? Interventions in the developed world (not in the context of depression) have been successful in effecting improvements in mother–infant interactions and infant attachment when addressing difficulties in parenting behaviors (Bakermans-Kranenburg, Van Ijzendoorn, & Juffer, 2003). It has, however, become clear that interventions principally directed at improving mother–infant interactions do not necessarily lead to improvements in maternal depression (Nylen, Moran, Franklin, & O'Hara, 2006), and treating maternal depression alone does not lead to improvements in child outcome (Forman et al., 2007). An additional concern is that health care resources are limited in the developing world, and consequently, interventions that capitalize upon locally available resources are a priority.

Several randomized controlled trials (RCTs) in developing contexts have demonstrated that psychological interventions delivered by local health workers may be helpful in reducing maternal depression and may have a positive impact upon some aspects of child development. In a large-scale RCT in rural Pakistan, a perinatal cognitive behavioral program delivered by primary care health workers, compared to enhanced usual care, halved rates of maternal depression (Rahman, Malik, Sikander, Roberts, & Creed, 2008). A reduction in maternal reports of rates of diarrhea and higher rates of completed courses of immunization were found, but no overall difference in infant growth. In an RCT in South Africa, examining an intervention specifically focused on the mother–infant relationship, Cooper et al. (2009) found a significant positive impact of their intervention, delivered by trained local women, on the quality of the mother–infant interactions and on security of infant attachment. No significant impact on maternal depressive disorder was found.

In another RCT conducted in Jamaica of a more general intervention targeting child rearing and parenting self-esteem, improvements were found in both maternal depressive symptoms (as measured by the CES-D) and infant global development in the treatment compared with the control group who received standard care (Baker-Henningham, Powell, Walker, & Grantham-McGregor, 2005). Again, the intervention was delivered by local community workers who were specifically trained. In India, community "participatory learning and action" groups, focused on education and maternal and newborn health practices led to a significant reduction in neonatal mortality rates (Tripathy et al., 2010). While the intervention was not targeted specifically at maternal depression, a reduction in moderate depression, as measured by the Kessler 10-item scale, was found in the intervention group compared with the control group in the third year after the start of the trial. Determining whether the improvements in the mother and infant outcomes are sustained over time will be an important question for future research.

CONCLUSION

Depression is a major contributor to the burden of disease in developing countries (Murray & Lopez, 1997). Postnatal depression is particularly important because it occurs at the time when both the mother and her rapidly developing infant are vulnerable to adverse effects in the environment. Prevalence studies have documented substantial rates of postnatal depression across many developing countries, with rates typically significantly higher than in developed contexts. Not only is an infant's development at increased risk of negative effects by the extreme levels of social and economic adversity often encountered in developing contexts, but it is likely to be further disrupted by the impact of postnatal depression on the quality of caregiving from the mother. There is compelling evidence linking postnatal depression to a raised risk for adverse infant outcomes in developed countries, and increasing evidence for a similar association in the developing world. Further, socioeconomic status has been shown to moderate the effects of postnatal depression on caregiving. It is, therefore, of paramount importance that interventions are developed and evaluated to support mothers and families in caring for young infants. There is a paucity of systematic intervention studies in developing compared to developed countries, but the available research suggests that mother–infant interactions and maternal depression should both be targets for treatment. Interventions that are sustainable and can be "scaled up" in developing countries with relatively limited resources are urgently required. The fact that such positive outcomes have been obtained in the RCTs to date using lay therapists is particularly promising in this regard. It should be emphasized that despite the adversity faced by mothers with depression and their infants in developing contexts, many children seem to remain physically healthy and develop normally, demonstrating remarkable resilience in both the quality of maternal caregiving and child development. One of the biggest issues facing clinicians and policy makers is the stigmatization of psychological problems. In order to support families with young children, where a caregiver is struggling with depression, it is essential that community-based interventions are readily available without stigma.

ACKNOWLEDGMENTS

We are grateful to Lynne Murray, Tamsen Rochat, and Linda Richter for their help in preparing the manuscript and to the Wellcome Trust, UK (grant 017571) and the TrygFonden Charitable Foundation for supporting this work.

REFERENCES

Adewuya, A. O., Ola, B. O., Aloba, O. O., Mapayi, B. M., & Okeniyi, J.A.O. (2008). Impact of postnatal depression on infants' growth in Nigeria. *Journal of Affective Disorders, 108*(1–2), 191–193.

Affonso, D. D., De, A. K., Horowitz, J. A., & Mayberry, L. J. (2000). An international study exploring levels of postpartum depressive symptomatology. *Journal of Psychosomatic Research, 49*(3), 207–216.

Agoub, M., Moussaoui, D., & Battas, O. (2005). Prevalence of postpartum depression in a Moroccan sample. *Archives of Women's Mental Health, 8*(1), 37–43.

Alkar, O. Y., & Gencoz, T. (2005). Critical factors associated with early postpartum depression among Turkish women. *Contemporary Family Therapy, 27*(2), 263–275.

Andajani-Sutjahjo, S., Manderson, L., & Astbury, J. (2007). Complex emotions, complex problems: Understanding the experiences of perinatal depression among new mothers in urban Indonesia. *Culture, Medicine, and Psychiatry, 31*(1), 101–122.

Anoop, S., Saravanan, B., Joseph, A., Cherian, A., & Jacob, K. S. (2004). Maternal depression and low maternal intelligence as risk factors for malnutrition in children: A community based case-control study from South India. *Archives of Disease in Childhood, 89*(4), 325–329.

Atkinson, L., Paglia, A., Coolbear, J., Niccols, A., Parker, K.C.H., & Guger, S. (2000). Attachment security: A meta-analysis of maternal mental health correlates. *Clinical Psychology Review, 20*(8), 1019–1040.

Avan, B., Ramchandani, P. G., Richter, L., Norris, S. A., & Stein, A. (2010). Maternal postnatal depression and children's growth and behaviour during the early years of life: Exploring the interaction between physical and mental health. *Archives of Disease in Childhood.*

Baggaley, R. F., Ganaba, R., Filippi, V., Kere, M., Marshall, T., Sombie, I., et al. (2007). Detecting depression after pregnancy: The validity of the K10 and K6 in Burkina Faso. *Tropical Medicine & International Health, 12*(10), 1225–1229.

Baker-Henningham, H., Powell, C., Walker, S., & Grantham-McGregor, S. (2003). Mothers of undernourished Jamaican children have poorer psychosocial functioning and this is associated with stimulation provided in the home. *European Journal of Clinical Nutrition, 57*(6), 786–792.

Baker-Henningham, H., Powell, C., Walker, S., & Grantham-McGregor, S. (2005). The effect of early stimulation on maternal depression: A cluster randomised controlled trial. *Archives of Disease in Childhood, 90*(12), 1230–1234.

Bakermans-Kranenburg, M. J., Van Ijzendoorn, M. H., & Juffer, F. (2003). Less is more: Meta-analyses of sensitivity and attachment interventions in early childhood. *Psychological Bulletin, 129*(2), 195–215.

Bamalingaswami, V., Jonsson, U., & Rohde, J. (1996). *Commentary on Nutrition, Progress of Nations.* New York: UNICEF.

Beck, C. T. (1996). A meta-analysis of predictors of postpartum depression. *Nursing Research, 45*(5), 297–303.

Black, M. M., Baqui, A. H., Zaman, K., Arifeen, S. E., & Black, R. E. (2009). Maternal depressive symptoms and infant growth in rural Bangladesh. *American Journal of Clinical Nutrition, 89*(3), 951S–957S.

Black, M. M., Walker, S. P., Wachs, T. D., Ulkuer, N., Gardner, J. M., Grantham-McGregor, S., et al. (2008). Policies to reduce undernutrition include child development. *The Lancet, 371*(9611), 454–455.

Boath, E. H., Pryce, A. J., & Cox, J. L. (1998). Postnatal depression: The impact on the family. *Journal of Reproductive and Infant Psychology, 16*(2–3), 199–203.

Broadhead, J. C., & Abas, M. A. (1998). Life events, difficulties and depression among women in an urban setting in Zimbabwe. *Psychological Medicine, 28*(1), 29–38.

Cattaneo, A., & Quintero-Romero, S. (2006). Protection, promotion and support of breastfeeding in low-income countries. *Seminars in Fetal and Neonatal Medicine, 11*(1), 48–53.

Chaaya, M., Campbell, O. M., El Kak, F., Shaar, D., Harb, H., & Kaddour, A. (2002). Postpartum depression: Prevalence and determinants in Lebanon. *Archives of Women's Mental Health, 5*(2), 65–72.

Chandran, M., Tharyan, P., Muliyil, J., & Abraham, S. (2002). Post-partum depression in a cohort of women from a rural area of Tamil Nadu, India: Incidence and risk factors. *British Journal of Psychiatry, 181*, 499–504.

Coleman, R., Morison, L., Paine, K., Powell, R. A., & Walraven, G. (2006). Women's reproductive health and depression: A community survey in the Gambia, West Africa. *Social Psychiatry Psychiatric Epidemiology, 41*(9), 720–727.

Cooper, P. J., Murray, L., & Stein, A. (1993). Psychosocial factors associated with the early termination of breast-feeding. *Journal of Psychosomatic Research, 37*(2), 171–176.

Cooper, P. J., Tomlinson, M., Swartz, L., Landman, M., Molteno, C., Stein, A., et al. (2009). Improving quality of mother–infant relationship and infant attachment in socioeconomically deprived community in South Africa: Randomised controlled trial. *British Medical Journal, 338*, b974.

Cooper, P. J., Tomlinson, M., Swartz, L., Woolgar, M., Murray, L., & Molteno, C. (1999). Post-partum depression and the mother–infant relationship in a South African peri-urban settlement. *British Journal of Psychiatry, 175*, 554–558.

De Miranda, C. T., Turecki, G., De Jesus Mari, J., Andreoli, S. B., Marcolim, M. A., Goihman, S., et al. (1996). Mental health of the mothers of malnourished children. *International Journal of Epidemiology, 25*(1), 128–133.

Dennis, C.L.E., Janssen, P. A., & Singer, J. (2004). Identifying women at-risk for postpartum depression in the immediate postpartum period. *Acta Psychiatrica Scandinavica, 110*(5), 338–346.

Evans, J., Heron, J., Patel, R. R., & Wiles, N. (2007). Depressive symptoms during pregnancy and low birth weight at term: Longitudinal study. *British Journal of Psychiatry, 191*, 84–85.

Falceto, O. G., Giugliani, E.R.J., & Fernandes, C.L.C. (2004). Influence of parental mental health on early termination of breast-feeding: A case-control study. *Journal of the American Board of Family Practice, 17*(3), 173–183.

Field, T., Diego, M., Dieter, J., Hernandez-Reif, M., Schanberg, S., & Kuhn, C. (2004). Prenatal depression effects on the fetus and the newborn. *Infant Behavior and Development, 27*(2), 216–229.

Fisher, J.R.W., Morrow, M. M., Ngoc, N.T.N., & Anh, L.T.H. (2004). Prevalence, nature, severity and correlates of postpartum depressive symptoms in Vietnam. *BJOG: An International Journal of Obstetrics and Gynaecology, 111*(12), 1353–1360.

Florenzano, R., Botto, A., Muniz, C., Rojas, J., Astorquiza, J., & Gutierrez, L. (2002). Frecuencia de sintomas depresivos medidos con el EPDS en puerperas hospitalizadas en el Hospital del Salvador. *Revista Chilena de neuropsiquiatria, 40*(4), 10.

Forman, D. R., O'Hara, M. W., Stuart, S., Gorman, L. L., Larsen, K. E., & Coy, K. C. (2007). Effective treatment for postpartum depression is not sufficient to improve the developing mother–child relationship. *Development and Psychopathology, 19*(2), 585–602.

Galler, J. R., Harrison, R. H., Biggs, M. A., Ramsey, F., & Forde, V. (1999). Maternal moods predict breastfeeding in Barbados. *Journal of Developmental and Behavioral Pediatrics, 20*(2), 80–87.

Galler, J. R., Harrison, R. H., Ramsey, F., Chawla, S., & Taylor, J. (2006). Postpartum feeding attitudes, maternal depression, and breastfeeding in Barbados. *Infant Behavior and Development, 29*(2), 189–203.

Galler, J. R., Harrison, R. H., Ramsey, F., Forde, V., & Butler, S. C. (2000). Maternal depressive symptoms affect infant cognitive development in Barbados. *Journal of Child Psychology and Psychiatry and Allied Disciplines, 41*(6), 747–757.

Gausia, K., Fisher, C., Ali, M., & Oosthuizen, J. (2009). Magnitude and contributory factors of postnatal depression: A community-based cohort study from a rural subdistrict of Bangladesh. *Psychological Medicine, 39*(6), 999–1007.

Glasser, S., Barell, V., Shoham, A., Ziv, A., Boyko, V., Lusky, A., et al. (1998). Prospective study of postpartum depression in an Israeli cohort: Prevalence, incidence and demographic risk factors. *Journal of Psychosomatic Obstetrics and Gynaecology, 19*(3), 155–164.

Grantham-McGregor, S., Cheung, Y. B., Cueto, S., Glewwe, P., Richter, L., & Strupp, B. (2007). Developmental potential in the first 5 years for children in developing countries. *The Lancet, 369*(9555), 60–70.

Hadley, C., Tegegn, A., Tessema, F., Asefa, M., & Galea, S. (2008). Parental symptoms of common mental disorders and children's social, motor, and language development in sub-Saharan Africa. *Annals of Human Biology, 35*(3), 259–275.

Harpham, T., Huttly, S., De Silva, M. J., & Abramsky, T. (2005). Maternal mental health and child nutritional status in four developing countries. *Journal of Epidemiology and Community Health, 59*(12), 1060–1064.

Henderson, J. J., Evans, S. F., Straton, J.A.Y., Priest, S. R., & Hagan, R. (2003). Impact of postnatal depression on breastfeeding duration. *Birth, 30*(3), 175–180.

Ho-Yen, S. D., Bondevik, G. T., Eberhard-Gran, M., & Bjorvatn, B. (2006). The prevalence of depressive symptoms in the postnatal period in Lalitpur district, Nepal. *Acta Obstetricia et Gynecologica Scandinavica, 85*(10), 1186–1192.

Husain, N., Bevc, I., Husain, M., Chaudhry, I. B., Atif, N., & Rahman, A. (2006). Prevalence and social correlates of postnatal depression in a low income country. *Archives of Women's Mental Health, 9*(4), 197–202.

Husain, N., Creed, F., & Tomenson, B. (2000). Depression and social stress in Pakistan. *Psychological Medicine, 30*(2), 395–402.

Kara, B., Ünalan, P., Çifçili, S., Cebeci, D. S., & Sarper, N. (2008). Is there a role for the family and close community to help reduce the risk of postpartum depression in new mothers? A cross-sectional study of Turkish women. *Maternal and Child Health Journal, 12*(2), 155–161.

Kirpinar, I., Gozum, S., & Pasinliolu, T. (2010). Prospective study of postpartum depression in eastern Turkey prevalence, socio-demographic and obstetric correlates, prenatal anxiety and early awareness. *Journal of Clinical Nursing, 19*(3–4), 422–431.

Kotchick, B. A., Forehand, R., Brody, G., Armistead, L., Simon, P., Morse, E., et al. (1997). The impact of maternal HIV infection on parenting in inner-city African American families. *Journal of Family Psychology, 11*(4), 447–461.

Kwalombota, M. (2002). The effect of pregnancy in HIV-infected women. *AIDS Care—Psychological and Socio-Medical Aspects of AIDS/HIV, 14*(3), 431–433.

Lawrie, T. A., Hofmeyr, G. J., De Jager, M., & Berk, M. (1998). Validation of the Edinburgh Postnatal Depression Scale on a cohort of South African women. *South African Medical Journal, 88*(10), 1340–1344.

Liabsuetrakul, T., Vittayanont, A., & Pitanupong, J. (2007). Clinical applications of anxiety, social support, stressors, and self-esteem measured during pregnancy and postpartum for screening postpartum depression in Thai women. *Journal of Obstetrics and Gynaecology Research, 33*(3), 333–340.

Lovestone, S., & Kumar, R. (1993). Postnatal psychiatric illness: The impact on partners. *British Journal of Psychiatry, 163*, 210–216.

Mahmud, W.M.R.W., Shariff, S., & Yaacob, M. J. (2002). Postpartum depression: A survey of the incidence and associated risk factors among Malay women in Meris Kubor Besar, Bachok, Kelantan. *Malaysian Journal of Medical Sciences, 9*(1), 41–48.

Marmot, M. (2010). *Fair society, healthy lives—The Marmot Review final report.* London: Department of Health.

Medhin, G., Hanlon, C., Dewey, M., Alem, A., Tesfaye, F., Worku, B., et al. (2010). Prevalence and predictors of undernutrition among infants aged six and twelve months in Butajira, Ethiopia: The P-MaMiE Birth Cohort. *BMC Public Health, 10,* 27.

Murray, C., & Lopez, A. D. (1997). Global mortality, disability, and the contribution of risk factors: Global burden of disease study. *The Lancet, 349*(9063), 1436–1442.

Murray, L., Halligan, S. L., & Cooper, P. J. (2010). Effects of postnatal depression on mother–infant interactions, and child development. In T. Wachs & G. Bremner (Eds.), *Handbook of infant development* (pp. 192–220. Hoboken, NJ: Wiley-Blackwell.

Nakku, J.E.M., Nakasi, G., & Mirembe, F. (2006). Postpartum major depression at six weeks in primary health care: Prevalence and associated factors. *African Health Sciences, 6*(4), 207–214.

Nhiwatiwa, S., Patel, V., & Acuda, W. (1998). Predicting postnatal mental disorder with a screening questionnaire: A prospective cohort study from Zimbabwe. *Journal of Epidemiology and Community Health, 52*(4), 262–266.

Nylen, K. J., Moran, T. E., Franklin, C. L., & O'Hara, M. W. (2006). Maternal depression: A review of relevant treatment approaches for mothers and infants. *Infant Mental Health Journal, 27*(4), 327–343.

O'Hara, M. W., & Swain, A. M. (1996). Rates and risk of postpartum depression—A meta-analysis. *International Review of Psychiatry, 8*(1), 37–54.

Owoeye, A. O., Aina, O. F., & Morakinyo, O. (2006). Risk factors of postpartum depression and EPDS scores in a group of Nigerian women. *Tropical Doctor, 36*(2), 100–103.

Patel, V., DeSouza, N., & Rodrigues, M. (2003). Postnatal depression and infant growth and development in low income countries: A cohort study from Goa, India. *Archives of Disease in Childhood, 88*(1), 34–37.

Patel, V., & Prince, M. (2006). Maternal psychological morbidity and low birth weight in India. *British Journal of Psychiatry, 188,* 284–285.

Pollock, J. I., Manaseki-Holland, S., & Patel, V. (2009). Depression in Mongolian women over the first 2 months after childbirth: Prevalence and risk factors. *Journal of Affective Disorders, 116*(1–2), 126–133.

Rahman, A., Bunn, J., Lovel, H., & Creed, F. (2007a). Association between antenatal depression and low birthweight in a developing country. *Acta Psychiatrica Scandinavica, 115*(6), 481–486.

Rahman, A., Bunn, J., Lovel, H., & Creed, F. (2007b). Maternal depression increases infant risk of diarrhoeal illness: A cohort study. *Archives of Disease in Childhood, 92*(1), 24–28.

Rahman, A., Harrington, R., & Bunn, J. (2002). Can maternal depression increase infant risk of illness and growth impairment in developing countries? *Child: Care, Health and Development, 28*(1), 51–56.

Rahman, A., Iqbal, Z., Bunn, J., Lovel, H., & Harrington, R. (2004). Impact of maternal depression on infant nutritional status and illness: A cohort study. *Archives of General Psychiatry, 61*(9), 946–952.

Rahman, A., Lovel, H., Bunn, J., Iqbal, Z., & Harrington, R. (2004). Mothers' mental health and infant growth: A case-control study from Rawalpindi, Pakistan. *Child: Care, Health and Development, 30*(1), 21–27.

Rahman, A., Malik, A., Sikander, S., Roberts, C., & Creed, F. (2008). Cognitive behaviour therapy–based intervention by community health workers for mothers with depression and their infants in rural Pakistan: A cluster-randomised controlled trial. *The Lancet, 372*(9642), 902–909.

Robertson, E., Grace, S., Wallington, T., & Stewart, D. E. (2004). Antenatal risk factors for postpartum depression: A synthesis of recent literature. *General Hospital Psychiatry, 26*(4), 289–295.

Rochat, T. J., Richter, L. M., Doll, H. A., Buthelezi, N. P., Tomkins, A., & Stein, A. (2006). Depression among pregnant rural South African women undergoing HIV testing. *Journal of the American Medical Association, 295*(12), 1376–1378.

Shonkoff, J. P., Boyce, W. T., & McEwen, B. S. (2009). Neuroscience, molecular biology, and the childhood roots of health disparities: Building a new framework for health promotion and disease prevention. *Journal of the American Medical Association, 301*(21), 2252–2259.

Smith, L. C., & Haddad, L. (2000). Explaining child malnutrition in developing countries: A cross-country analysis. *Research Report of the International Food Policy Research Institute, 111*, 1–112.

Stein, A., Gath, D. H., Bucher, J., Bond, A., Day, A., & Cooper, P. J. (1991). The relationship between post-natal depression and mother–child interaction. *British Journal of Psychiatry, 158*, 46–52.

Stein, A., Krebs, G., Richter, L., Tomkins, A., Rochat, T., & Bennish, M. L. (2005). Babies of a pandemic. *Archives of Disease in Childhood, 90*(2), 116–118.

Stein, A., Malmberg, L. E., Sylva, K., Barnes, J., Leach, P., & Team, F.C.C.C. (2008). The influence of maternal depression, caregiving, and socioeconomic status in the post-natal year on children's language development. *Child: Care, Health and Development, 34*(5), 603–612.

Stewart, R. C., Bunn, J., Vokhiwa, M., Umar, E., Kauye, F., Fitzgerald, M., et al. (2010). Common mental disorder and associated factors amongst women with young infants in rural Malawi. *Social Psychiatry and Psychiatric Epidemiology, 45*(5), 551–559.

Stewart, R. C., Umar, E., Kauye, F., Bunn, J., Vokhiwa, M., Fitzgerald, M., et al. (2008). Maternal common mental disorder and infant growth: A cross-sectional study from Malawi. *Maternal and Child Nutrition, 4*(3), 209–219.

Surkan, P. J., Kawachi, I., & Peterson, K. E. (2008). Childhood overweight and maternal depressive symptoms. *Journal of Epidemiology and Community Health, 62*(5), e11.

Surkan, P. J., Kawachi, I., Ryan, L. M., Berkman, L. F., Vieira, L.M.C., & Peterson, K. E. (2008). Maternal depressive symptoms, parenting self-efficacy, and child growth. *American Journal of Public Health, 98*(1), 125–132.

Taj, R., & Sikander, K. S. (2003). Effects of maternal depression on breastfeeding. *Journal of Pakistan Medical Association, 53*(1), 8–11.

Tesfaye, M., Hanlon, C., Wondimagegn, D., & Alem, A. (2010). Detecting postnatal common mental disorders in Addis Ababa, Ethiopia: Validation of the Edinburgh Postnatal Depression Scale and Kessler Scales. *Journal of Affective Disorders, 122*(1–2), 102–108.

Tomlinson, M., Cooper, P., & Murray, L. (2005). The mother–infant relationship and infant attachment in a South African peri-urban settlement. *Child Development, 76*(5), 1044–1054.

Tomlinson, M., Cooper, P. J., Stein, A., Swartz, L., & Molteno, C. (2006). Postpartum depression and infant growth in a South African peri-urban settlement. *Child: Care, Health and Development, 32*(1), 81–86.

Tripathy, P., Nair, N., Barnett, S., Mahapatra, R., Borghi, J., Rath, S., et al. (2010). Effect of a participatory intervention with women's groups on birth outcomes and maternal depression in Jharkhand and Orissa, India: A cluster-randomised controlled trial. *The Lancet, 375*(9721), 1182–1192.

UNICEF. (1998). *State of the world's children 1998*. New York.

Walker, S. P., Wachs, T. D., Meeks Gardner, J., Lozoff, B., Wasserman, G. A., Pollitt, E., et al. (2007). Child development: Risk factors for adverse outcomes in developing countries. *The Lancet, 369*(9556), 145–157.

Wang, S. Y., Jiang, X. Y., Jan, W. C., & Chen, C. H. (2003). A comparative study of postnatal depression and its predictors in Taiwan and mainland China. *American Journal of Obstetrics and Gynecology, 189*(5), 1407–1412.

Weissman, M. M., Leaf, P. J., Tischler, G. L., Blazer, D. G., Karno, M., Bruce, M. L., et al. (1988). Affective disorders in five United States communities. *Psychological Medicine, 18*(1), 141–153.

Wilson, L. M., Reid, A. J., Midmer, D. K., Biringer, A., Carroll, J. C., & Stewart, D. E. (1996). Antenatal psychosocial risk factors associated with adverse postpartum family outcomes. *Canadian Medical Association Journal, 154*(6), 785–798.

Wolf, A. W., De Andraca, I., & Lozoff, B. (2002). Maternal depression in three Latin American samples. *Social Psychiatry and Psychiatric Epidemiology, 37*(4), 169–176.

World Health Organization. (1995). *Physical status: The use and interpretation of anthropometry. Report of a WHO Expert Committee*. Geneva, Switzerland.

World Health Organization. (2000). *Global water supply and sanitation assessment*. Geneva, Switzerland.

World Health Organization. (2003). *Global strategy for infant and young child feeding*. Geneva, Switzerland.

Chapter 5

WITHDRAWAL BEHAVIOR AND DEPRESSION IN INFANCY

Antoine Guedeney and Kaija Puura

With the Baby Alarm Distress Scale Study Group (Monica Oliver, Argentina; Daphna Dollberg, Israel; Simone Facuri-Lopes, Brazil; Mirjami Mäntymaa, Finland; Stephen Matthey, Jennifer Re, and Samuel Menahem, Australia; Barbara Figueiredo, Joana Silva, and Isobel Soares, Portugal; Emilia de Rosa, Italy; Lisa Milne, Australia; Vibeke Moe, Unni Tranaas Vannebo, Kari Slinning, Hanne Braarud, and Lars Smith, Norway; Mikael Heinmann, Sweden; Dora Musetti, Uruguay; Jorge Tizon, Spain; J. Wendland and B. Grollemund, France)

Social and emotional development in early infancy is widely recognized as crucial for all aspects of functioning throughout the lifespan (Sroufe, 1995). The infant's ability to relate to and understand the social world develops within the close and continuous interactions between parent and infant. Several factors can have a deleterious effect on early infant social and emotional development. Social risk factors include infant prematurity or illness, genetic risk factors, living in inadequate or inappropriately stimulating environments, and early disruptions in the parent–child relationship and the adequacy of parental care (Feldman, 2007). Parental mental illness also poses a risk for infant attachment and social and emotional development (Field, 2001; Murray, Fiori-Cowley,

---

A former version of this chapter was made for the Lars Sven jubilee, to be published in Norwegian, along with Kajia Puura, Mirjami Mäntymaa, and Tuula Tamminen. Published with permission.

Hooper, & Cooper, 1996; Teti, Gelfand, Messinger, & Isabella, 1995). The influence of potential risk factors on infant development is dependent on qualities of both the parent and of the infant, which together determine the mutual adaptation capacity of the dyad (Mäntymaa, 2006), and its capacity to develop a parent-infant synchrony within the first 18 months of life of the infant (Feldman, 2007).

INFANT DEPRESSION: DOES IT EXIST?

Infant depression was a starting point in the history of infant psychiatry (Guedeney, 2007). We use the term infant depression often, and this label brings with it the recognition of the infant as a person, of being someone who can suffer psychic pain. Depression in older children and adults is seen as the psychological survival mechanism in face of unbearable situation, where an individual loses his or her interest in interacting with the world and his or her emotions get flattened. Using the term depression with infants then means that the infant also has tried all solutions for keeping his balance. Even though we use the word often, we know very little about infant depression. We don't know when it begins. Can depression in infancy have an onset at any age, or is there an age limit? What do we actually call depression in infancy, between zero and three years of age? On the model of DSM-IV there is a recent tendency to diagnose major depressive disorder very early in life, as early as two and a half to three years. However, the proposal here is that there are no major depression disorders developing before three years of age, or two and a half at the earliest (Guedeney, 2007). Before that limit, the suggestion is to use the concept of sustained withdrawal behavior, described by Engel and Reischman (1956, 1979), *a propos* of the famous case of Monica. The learned helplessness paradigm (Seligman, Abramson, Semmel, & von Baeyer, 1979) may prove useful for understanding what kind of relationship leads to infant depression. There might be a continuum between withdrawal reaction and infant depression, withdrawal being a first level of reaction of an infant trapped in an inescapable situation (Guedeney, 2007).

The DC 0–3R (Zero to Three, 1995) classification system places infant depression into the affective disorders, and the revised version (DC: 0–3R) of the diagnostic system includes more detailed criteria for major depression in infancy. These criteria are based on the Research Diagnostic Criteria Revision (RDC-R, AACAP) and this gives a much more precise description and inclusion criteria for depression in toddlers. We now have Luby's proposals for adaptation to children aged two to five years (Luby et al., 2006). With these criteria she finds that 33% of 3- to 5.6-year-old children in a clinical community sample could have major depression. But this leads to the risk of clear over diagnosis. Why should depression be more frequent in early childhood that later on, even in a community referred sample?

ANIMAL MODELS OF DEPRESSION
AND WITHDRAWAL

Bowlby has described attachment and withdrawal systems as distinct, though having the same function, and triggered by the same situations, and (both system) easily conflicting (Bowlby, 1973). Panksepp has proposed a schema of the main types of emotional systems in mammalians: lust, care, panic, play, fear, rage, and seeking in which withdrawal behavior appears to be part of the panic and fear systems (Panksepp, 2006). Therefore, withdrawal behavior is clearly recognized as a behavioral and emotional system in infants.

The link between depression/withdrawal reaction in infants and learned helplessness behavior was made relatively recently. In the famous, but now ethically disputable experimentation by Seligman et al. in 1979, a dog was electrically shocked in an inescapable situation. This situation they called the learned helplessness situation, which lead in the dog to resignation. The model of learned helplessness has become a model for depression, and to the use of the learned helplessness paradigm as a key screening test for antidepressant activity (Seligman et al., 1979). Some recent advances in veterinary medicine are fascinating for us, infancy mental health professionals: It is now possible to describe a nosography of attachment-based behavioral disorders in dogs and cats (Pageat, 1995). Clearly, infant mental health professionals are interested in the richness and complexity of clinical syndromes of depression in puppies and kittens, as they provide us both with clear cut physiopathological, evolution and therapeutic frameworks for different kind of clinical situations related to depression, attachment disorders, separation anxiety and phobias (Pageat, 1995).

The concept of approach/withdrawal seems to be fundamental in the analysis of behavioral development (Greenberg, 1995). Comparative psychology could help screen the pathways of this behavior and to look for the genes implicated in this endophenotype, particularly around dopamine and DRD4 alleles, since such correlations have been found for the genetic susceptibility of attachment disorganization (Bakermans-Kranenburg & van IJzendoorn, 2007). An endophenotype is a measurable component unseen by the unaided eye along the pathway between disease and distal genotype. It may be neurophysiological, or biochemical, or neuropsychological in nature. Endophenotypes represent simpler clues to genetic underpinning than the disease syndrome itself (Gottesman & Gould, 2003).

WITHDRAWAL BEHAVIOR IN INFANTS

The term *withdrawal* has been known and used in the clinical study of infancy, although it is hard to find a clear definition of it. Clinical reports and research findings on the subject are surprisingly rare. To some extent withdrawal is a normal feature of parent–infant interaction and plays an important role in its regulation (Brazelton, Koslowski, & Main, 1974). Engel and Reichsman (1956) described pathological withdrawal in a marasmic and developmentally retarded infant, Monica, who came to their pediatric service with severe failure to thrive (FTT) when she was 14 months old. She had esophageal atresia and required feeding through a gastric fistula. When her care was abruptly transferred from her warm grandmother to her isolated mother, who was disgusted by her fistula, she was noted to withdraw, cry, and lose weight although no physical cause was found. Now she would probably be considered as a typical case of disorganized attachment. After prolonged care, she improved and developed normally.

More recently, based on extended clinical experience, Fraiberg (1980, 1982) described a group of pathological defenses observed between 3 and 18 months of age in infants who experienced severe danger and deprivation. These early defenses, "avoidance," "freezing," and "fighting," are, following Selma Fraiberg, apparently summoned from a biological repertoire. Thus, withdrawal takes an important place, both in physiology and in pathology, in the infant's repertoire of response to stress. Infant withdrawal appears also to be a key symptom of infant depression, as it seems unlikely that a depressed infant show no sign of withdrawal; however, withdrawal reaction appears to cover a much larger scope than infant depression, including attachment disorders, autistic syndromes, post traumatic stress syndrome and anxiety. A sustained withdrawal reaction can also be observed in many acute and chronic organic conditions. In between, intense and chronic pain in infancy is characterized by a very severe withdrawal reaction that correlates with the intensity of the pain (Gauvain-Piquard, Rodary, Rezvani, & Serbouti, 1999).

Sustained withdrawal reaction seems to be a good target for early screening in infant mental health, as negative symptoms are more difficult to assess than the more obvious, positive ones, and because withdrawal is a major component in the infant's behavioral response repertoire to stress and relationship disorders; moreover, this behavior has to be assessed within a relationship established with the child (Guedeney, 1997). Feldman stresses the importance of withdrawal behavior in infants as a sign of a dysregulation of parent–infant synchrony (Mäntymaa, 2006; Feldman, 2007).

MATERNAL DEPRESSION, MATERNAL ANXIETY, INFANT DEPRESSION, AND WITHDRAWAL

The relationship between maternal and infant depression is no more direct or simple than the one between separation and depression in infants. The infant's reactions to the interruption or to the violation of the expectations within the interaction are both obvious and durable in the still-face paradigm (Cohn & Tronick, 1983), or in the experimental desynchronization setting designed by Murray and Trevarthen (1986). The infant's reaction to these different conditions follows a path clearly delineated by Robertson and Bowlby (1952), with the key sequence of surprise, protestation, withdrawal, and despair. Tronick has recently insisted on the effect of maternal depression on the extension of what he calls the *dyadic states of consciousness* (Tronick & Weinberg, 1997). These key studies have shown some possible models of transmission of the depressive affect between mother and child, using the still face paradigm. Depressed mothers are less positive and more negative when interacting with their infants. Infants of depressed mothers are less positive and more negative when interacting with their mothers in these laboratory situations. More to the point is the fact that infants of depressed mothers show depressed behavior even with nondepressed adults, demonstrating a generalization of the depressive model of the relationship (Field, 2001; Field et al., 1988; Field, Diego, Hernandez-Reif, & Fernandez, 2007; Field et al., 2006). These behaviors result at least in part from the poorer interaction provided by the mother, as postpartum depressed mothers have been observed for instance to be less contingent and less affectively attuned to their infant (Murray et al., 1996).

Postpartal interaction may not be the only way maternal depression and anxiety affect the development of the infant. Several studies have suggested that both mother's anxiety and depression during gestation have a negative effect on the fetus behavior and development: fetuses of anxious/depressed pregnant women show signs of behavioral immaturity when compared with fetus of nonanxious/nondepressed pregnant women (DiPietro, Hilton, Hawkins, Costigan, & Pressman, 2002). It has also been shown that mothers of newborn infants with poorer motor maturity are particularly at risk to develop postpartum depression, and also that new-borns of mothers depressed at delivery are less socially competent before even interacting with their mothers (Hernandez-Reif, Field, Diego, & Ruddock, 2006). This does not mean that infant's withdrawal is a passive behavior, a simple imitation of the mother's behavior. On the contrary, the depressive state of the infant is in no way a pure biological reaction, but a defensive organization of its own. Children of mothers reporting being more depressed or anxious since childbirth obtain significantly higher Baby Alarm Distress Scale (ADBB) scores (Matthey, Guedeney, Starakis, & Barnett, 2005), using Cox, Holden, and Sagovsky's EPDS scale (Cox, Holden, and Sagovsky, 1987); and children evaluated with higher values of social withdrawal show less optimal behavior in the interaction with their mothers (Dollberg, Feldman, Keren, & Guedeney, 2006; Puura, Guedeney, Mantymaa, & Tamminen, 2007).

THE ASSESSMENT OF SUSTAINED WITHDRAWAL REACTION IN INFANTS: THE DEVELOPMENT OF THE BABY ALARM DISTRESS SCALE

It is most important to identify infant withdrawal behavior as an alarm distress symptom before it becomes obvious (Ironside, 1975). Despite the formidable developmental changes in the course of infancy, it seems possible to assess a sustained withdrawal reaction in infants anywhere between 2 and 24 months of age, provided the duration of the with-drawal and its persistence in different types of relationships is checked. The ADBB (Guedeney & Fermanian, 2001) was initially designed to fit with the medical examination in a well-baby clinic. It was used here as was Winnicott's set "situation" (Winnicott, 1941) providing a somewhat regularly defined stimulation and observing the way the infant makes use of it. However, any other structured situations can be used to assess with-drawal behavior, for instance, or the still face, or the strange situation, or a Crowell assessment situation. The advantage of the scale is that it assesses infant social behavior with a stranger, rather than using the caregiver who may feel pressure to perform if asked to interact with her infant during an observation and requires no special equipment (Matthey et al., 2005). The scale has eight items, rated zero to four, with zero being normal and 32 the maximum score. The ADBB is a clinical instrument aimed at evalu-ating social behaviors that can be easily observed during a brief observa-tion among children 2–24 months old. These behaviors are organized into eight items/categories: (1) Facial Expression, (2) Eye Contact, (3) Gen-eral Level of Activity, (4) Self-Stimulating Gestures, (5) Vocalizations,

(6) Response to Stimulation, (7) Relationship, and (8) Attraction. Each item is rated from 0 to 4 (0 = no unusual behavior; 4 = severe unusual behavior) and a trained observer only needs an observation of 10 to 15 minutes in order to score the ADBB details and translations in several languages can be found on the ADBB Web site (http://www.adbb.net/), as well as the manual for use.

The scale has been used in different studies in Argentina, Armenia, Australia, Brazil, Finland, France, Israel, Italy, Norway, Portugal, South Africa, and Spain, with different kind of population and settings and different methodologies. An important point about the transcultural validity is that five studies found the same cut off score of 5 and over, in France, Finland, Israel, Italy, and Brazil. However, an ongoing study in Norway indicates that a lower threshold (4) might be interesting for screening (Heimann et al., unpublished manuscript). The scale has been shown to have good reliability and validity (Matthey et al., 2005). Subsequent research has shown the factor structure to vary across samples and further research has been recommended (Matthey et al., 2005). To test the clinical validity of the scale, Dollberg et al. (2006) compared a group of clinic-referred infants with a control group and found that ADBB scores were significantly higher in the clinic-referred group. The mothers of the withdrawn infants were observed to be more intrusive, the infants were less involved in the relationship and there was generally lower reciprocity in the mother–infant relationship. Mothers in the referred group were more depressed, which in turn was associated with poorer relational patterns in both the mother and the child (Dollberg et al., 2006). Gender differences were also noted, with girls being less prone to a withdrawal response. One Finnish study (Puura et al., 2010) gave the first estimation of the prevalence of withdrawal behavior at different ages, taking advantage of the Finnish well-baby clinics network used by more than 90% of the families. The aims of the study were to see whether an infant observation method can be used reliably by front line workers in primary health care, and to examine the prevalence of infants' social withdrawal symptoms. A random sample of 491 parents with 4-, 8-, or 18-month-old infants was asked to participate in the study. Parents of 363 infants (74%) agreed to participate. The infants were examined by general practitioners (GPs) during routine checkups in well-baby clinics and their withdrawal symptoms were assessed with the ADBB. A score of 5 or more on the ADBB scale in two subsequent assessments at a two-week interval was regarded as a sign of clinically significant infant social withdrawal. The ADBB scale proved to be a feasible and reliable method for detecting infant social withdrawal. Approximately 3% of infants were showing social withdrawal as a sign of distress in this normal population sample. Another Finnish study showed the importance of looking for maternal depression and paternal mental health disorders if an infant is found to be withdrawn (Mäntymaa, Puura, Kaukonen, Salmelin, & Tamminen, 2008).

A study by Figueiredo in Portugal showed that the scale was very sensitive to change, in a sample of infants of young adolescent mothers being depressed (Figueiredo, Bifulco, Pacheco, Costa, & Magarinho, 2006); a more recent study showed links between prenatal anxiety and depression and ulterior withdrawal behavior in the child (Figueiredo et al., under review). Matthey, Crncec, and Guedeney have developed a short version of the ADBB (M-ADBB), to be used as a screening tool in the Australian context, but which still waits for further validation. This version, the *modified ADBB*, includes only five areas: (1) Facial Expression, (2) Eye Contact, (3) Vocalization, (4) Activity Level, and (5) Relationship. In addition, the scoring is changed to three global levels: no problem, possible problem area, and definite problem area. Matthey and Crncec are currently making studies on the training and inter rater reliability of both scales, ADBB and M-ADBB. A recently published study using the m-ADBB (Hartley et al., 2010) showed a high rate of withdrawal with HIV-positive infants from HIV-positive mothers in South Africa.

Two studies in France have confirmed the validity of the scale, on top of the original validation study (Guedeney & Fermanian, 2001), on a sample of 64 well-baby clinic infants aged 2–24 months. The first one was made in Lyon, with 54 nonclinical dyads followed using clinical assessment, ADBB, EPDS and an interaction al measure of the quality of parent child play, PIPE. The study showed that assessing withdrawal behavior using three measures at different ages (3, 6, and 12 months) allowed for a good screening of mother child interactional disorders (Rochette & Mellier, 2007). The second study was made in Paris in a public screening health center, on 650 infants aged 10–18 months (Guedeney, Foucault, Bougen, Larroque, & Mentré, 2008) a total of 640 children with a mean age of 16 months were included in the study. Thirteen percent ($n = 85$) of the children had an ADBB score at 5 or over, and 8% ($n = 51$) of the infants had a score over 5. ADBB scores ranged from 0 to 19. There is a clear correlation between withdrawal behavior and the level of psychological difficulties as observed during the medical and psychological examination (29.6% vs. 9.6%) and between withdrawal and developmental delay (52.6% vs. 11.8%). Among withdrawn infants having psychological difficulties, 9.2% had sleep disorders, 5.3% had relational and behavioral difficulties and 3% had developmental delay disorders. More boys than girls were withdrawn (16.18% vs. 9.33%), more difficult family situations (joint custody or foster family): 35.7% vs. 12.1%,), more adopted children (57.1% vs. 12.5%), and more twins (37.5% vs. 12.5%). More withdrawn infants are taken care of at home (15.1% vs. 9.0%). No correlation was found between the SES level of the family, the ethnic origin of the child, gender, rank of birth, birth weight or prematurity, nor with any particular medical pathology, except for endocrine disorders and thriving difficulties. Another study is now being done, within the INSERM EDEN study of prenatal risk factors, including 1,000 infants assessed with the ADBB scale at one year. Two studies were made in day care setting with ADBB, one in Sao Paulo, Brazil (Assumpçao et al., 2000), and one in Paris (Guedeney, Grasso, & Starakis, 2004).

A recently launched project in Norway investigates how ADBB can be used in well-baby clinics in order to detect infants at risk for nonoptimal development (Heimann et al., submitted manuscript). The study follows 242 children from 3 to 12 months of age (192 children born at term; 50 children born 4 to 10 weeks prematurely). All children will be assessed three times with the ADBB (at three and nine months by a nurse and at six months by a GP). A follow-up at 12 months of age assesses the well-being of the mother and infant using checklists, questionnaires, interviews, and observations. Data collection starts in January 2008 and ends in October 2009. This study will assess the predictive validity of the scale, and its interest as a screening instrument in well-baby clinics. The purpose of the present study is to investigate if sustained withdrawal, as measured with a new instrument (ADBB), can be reliable evaluated during regular visits to well-baby clinic and if the information thus collected will give valuable information regarding the child's further psychosocial development. The study has a unique longitudinal design that will make it possible to investigate both stability over time and the impact of withdrawal reactions on individual developmental trajectories. In order to guarantee that the study includes children displaying a large enough variability in withdrawal reactions the sample will be divided in two different groups: One group of developing children born at term and one group prematurely born children. In addition, observed sustained withdrawal will be related to important family characteristics (depression, personality and parent–infant interactive style).

The scale has been validated in several countries and in different settings. Its face validity seems very good, as the scale is easy to use both in clinical practice and in research. However, training is necessary to reach reliability, and Matthey and Crncec have developed a training set of videos and manuals for both ADBB and M-ADBB. The Australian, Finnish, Argentinian, Brazilian (Facuri-Lopes, Ricas, & Cotta Mancini, 2008), and

Norwegian teams have developed quite an experience in training GPs, pediatricians and mental health professionals. The sensitivity and sensibility of the scale are good in all validations available, with good Cronbach alphas. The scale is fairly stable on test retest, as shown in the Paris validation. Confirmatory factor analysis in the Brazilian Lopes study show three factors, with item 5, autostimulating gestures, standing alone, along with the two hypothesized dimensions, interpersonal and noninterpersonal. No study so far has yielded a result that was going against literature or clinical expertise: withdrawal behavior in infants is not linked with ethnicity, with parent's age or SES, but is linked with every condition known to hamper parent child relationship or with the ability of the child to establish and sustain relationships. The study by Milne, Greenway, and Guedeney (2009) shows the predictive validity of the scale, as does the EDEN study (Larroque, submitted manuscript). This study provides two important contributions to the literature on infant withdrawal. Firstly, it documents the longer terms effects of infant withdrawal. Secondly, it provides data supporting the longer-term validity of the ADBB, thus emphasizing its importance as an early screening measure. The results clearly demonstrate that withdrawal in early infancy (about six months' age), as measured by the ADBB are associated with later behavioral and developmental functioning. As one might have predicted, the ADBB seems particularly sensitive to predicting later social and communication problems. Infants who showed signs of withdrawal later as toddlers tended to be rated as higher on the Social Skills subscale of the BASC-2 suggesting that they had more difficulty with the interpersonal aspects of social adaptation. Similarly, withdrawn infants later as toddlers showed poor communication in terms of their functional communication (the ability to express ideas and communicate in a way that others can understand (as measured by the BASC-2) and in terms of their formal expressive and receptive language skills, as independently assessed using the Bayley-III. Interestingly, infant withdrawal was only associated with two types of behavioral problems, as reported by the mother, atypicality and attention problems. Atypicality measures the tendency of the child to behave in odd or peculiar ways, as marked by their disconnection or lack of awareness of their surrounds. High scores on this scale may reflect psychotic or autistic disorders.

Recently, more research attention has been given to early identification of autism. However, most of the studies exploring early autistic features use young preschool age children, about two to three years of age. The finding of this study suggests that there is potentially some aspect of sustained withdrawal in infancy that may point to autistic spectrum disorders (hence, it is likely that that infant withdrawal resulting from an early impoverished mother–infant relationship results in inattention and possible learning difficulties in early toddlerhood).

The scale is interesting to use with premature infants, who are especially at risk of relationship disorders and of withdrawal behavior. Although sustained withdrawal behavior is a key symptom of the diagnostic of autism, to date, it has received little attention in studies of precursory signs of pervasive developmental disorders (PDD). The aim of the study by Wendland, Gautier, Wolff, Brisson, and Adrien (2010) was to identify early signs of sustained withdrawal behavior in infants, aged from birth to 18 months, later diagnosed as autistic, through the analysis of home movies. The validity of the ADBB in the screening of early signs of autism was tested by comparison with a specific scale of autistic behaviors in infants: the ECA-N. Compared to normal infants, infants with a PDD have higher and more lingering scores of sustained withdrawal behavior during their first 18 months. While infants with PDD showed important interindividual differences in the ADBB and the ECA-N assessments, their individual scores profiles in the ADBB and the ECA-N were very similar. The strong correlation between the scores of the ADBB and the ECA-N may confirm the potential predictive value of sustained withdrawal behavior in the screening of autism. However, sustained withdrawal behavior may not be present since the first months of life and may show important variability during the first 18 months.

CONCLUSION

One of the most important tasks in the field of infant psychopathology is to identify the kind of relationship disturbances that can be linked specifically with each diagnostic category, here infant depression, and to assess the developmental transformation of infant depression over time, particularly within periods of acute developmental transformation. Infant withdrawal behavior is an interesting endophenotype and a good alarm signal. More studies are needed to link withdrawal with genetic susceptibility, particularly with the DRD4 alleles, to address infants with special needs and specific risk situation (as clef palate abnormalities) and to assess the efficiency of training with the ADBB.

REFERENCES

Assupmçao, F. B., Kuczynski, E., Gabriel Da Silva Gego, M., & Castanho de Almeida Rocca, C. (2000). Escala de avaliaçao da retraçao no bebê: um estudo de validade. *Archivos de Neuro-psiquiatria, 60,* 56–60.

Bakermans-Kranenburg, M. J., & van IJzendoorn, M. H. (2007). Research review: Genetic vulnerability or differential susceptibility in child development: The case of attachment. *Journal of Child Psychology and Psychiatry, 48,* 1160–1173.

Bowlby, J. (1973). *Attachment and loss* (Vol. 2). New York: Basic Books.

Brazelton, T. B., Koslowski, B., & Main, M. (1974). Origins of reciprocity. In M. Lewis & L. Rosenblum (Eds.), *Mother infant interaction* (pp. 57–70). New York: John Wiley.

Cohn, J. F., & Tronick, E. Z. (1983). Three month old infant's reaction to simulated maternal depression. *Child Development, 54,* 334–235.

Cox, J. L., Holden, J. M., & Sagovsky, R. (1987). Detection of postnatal depression: Development of the 10-item Edinburgh Depression Scale. *British Journal of Psychiatry, 150,* 782–786.

DiPietro, J. A., Hilton, S. C., Hawkins, M., Costigan, K. A., & Pressman, E. K. (2002). Maternal stress and affect influence fetal neurobehavioral development. *Developmental Psychology, 38*(5), 659–668.

Dollberg, D., Feldman, R., Keren, M., Guedeney, A. (2006). Sustained withdrawal behavior in clinic referred and nonreferred infants. *Infant Mental Health Journal, 27*(3), 292–309.

Engel, G. L., & Reichsman, F. (1956). Spontaneous and experimentally induced depression in an infant with gastric fistula: A contribution to the problem of depression. *Journal of the American Psychoanalytical Association, 4,* 428–452.

Engel, G. L., & Reichsman, F. (1979). Monica: A 25 years follow-up longitudinal study of the consequences of trauma in infancy. *Journal of the American Psychoanalytical Association, 27,* 107–126.

Facuri-Lopes, S., Ricas, J., & Cotta Mancini, M. (2008). Evaluation of the psychometric properties of the alarm distress baby scale among 122 Brazilian children. *Infant Mental Health Journal, 29,* 153–173.

Feldman, R. (2007). Parent-infant synchrony and the construction of shared timing; physiological precursors, developmental outcomes, and risk conditions. *Journal of Child Psychology and Psychiatry, 48,* 329–354.

Field, T. (2001). Chronic maternal depression affects infants, newborns and the fetus. In S. Goodman (Ed.), *Children of depressed parents: Alternative pathways and risk for psychopathology,* 59–88. Mahwah, NJ: Lawrence Erlbaum Associates.

Field, T., Diego, M., Hernandez-Reif, M., & Fernandez, M. (2007). Depressed mothers' newborns show less discrimination of other newborns' cry sounds. *Infant Behaviour and Development, 30*(3), 431–435.

Field, T., Healy, B., Goldstein, S., Perry, S., Bendell, D., Schanberg, S., et al. (1988). Infants of depressed mothers show "depressed" behavior even with nondepressed adults. *Child Development, 59*(6), 1569–1579.

Field, T., Hernandez-Reif, M., Diego, M., Figueiredo, B., Schanberg, S., & Kuhn, C. (2006). Prenatal cortisol, prematurity and low birthweight. *Infant Behavior and Development, 29,* 268–275.

Figueiredo, B., Bifulco, A., Pacheco, A., Costa, R., & Magarinho, R. (2006). Teenage pregnancy, attachment style and depression: A comparison of teenage and adult pregnant women in a Portuguese series. *Attachment and Human Development, 8*(2), 123–138.

Fraiberg, S. (1980). *Clinical studies in infant mental health: The first year of life.* London: Tavistock.

Fraiberg, S. (1982). Pathological defences in infancy. *Psychoanalytical Quarterly, 4,* 612–635.

Gauvain-Piquard, A., Rodary, C., Rezvani, A., & Serbouti, S. (1999). The development of the DEGR: A scale to assess pain in young children with cancer. *European Journal of Pain, 3,* 165–176.

Gottesman I. I., & Gould, T. D. (2003). The endophenotype concept in psychiatry: Ethymology and strategic intentions. *American Journal of Psychiatry, 160*(4), 636–645.

Greenberg, G. (1995). The historical development of the approach/withdrawal concept. In K. E. Hood, G. Greenberg, & E. Tobach (Eds.), *Behavioural development: Concepts of approach/withdrawal and integrative levels* (pp. 3–18). New York: Garland.

Guedeney, A. (1997). From early withdrawal reaction to infant depression: A baby alone does exist. *Infant Mental Health Journal, 18,* 339–349.

Guedeney, A. (2007). Infant's withdrawal and depression. *Infant Mental Health Journal, 28,* 399–408.

Guedeney, A., & Fermanian, J. (2001). A validity and reliability study of assessment and screening for sustained withdrawal reaction in infancy: The alarm distress baby scale. *Infant Mental Health Journal, 22*(5), 559–575.

Guedeney, A., Foucault, C., Bougen, E., Larroque, B., & Mentré, F. (2008). Screening for risk factors of relational withdrawal behaviour in infants aged 14–18 months. *European Psychiatry, 23,* 150–155.

Guedeney, A., Grasso, F., & Strarakis, N. (2004). Le séjour en crèche des jeunes enfants: Sécurité de l'attachement, tempérament et fréquence des maladies. *La Psychiatrie del enfant, 47,* 259–312.

Hartley, C., Pretorius, K., Mohammed, I., Laughton, B., Mahdi, S., Cotton, M. I., et al. (2010). Maternal postpartum depression and infant social withdrawal among immunodeficiency virus (HIV) positive mother–infant dyads. *Psychology, Health & Medicine, 15,* 278–287.

Hernandez-Reif, M., Field, T., Diego, M., & Ruddock, M. (2006). Greater arousal and less attentiveness to face/voice stimuli by neonates of depressed mothers on the Brazelton Neonatal Behavioral Assessment Scale. *Infant Behavior and Development, 29,* 594–598.

Ironside, W. (1975). The Infant Development Distress (IDD) syndrome: A predictor of impaired development? *Australian and New Zealand Journal of Psychiatry, 9,* 153–158.

Luby, J. L., Sullivan, J., Belden, A., Stalets, M., Blankenship, S., & Spitznagel, E. (2006). An observational analysis of behavior in depressed preschoolers: Further validation of early-onset depression. *Journal of the American Academy of Child and Adolescent Psychiatry, 45*, 203–212.

Mäntymaa, M. (2006). *Early mother–infant interaction: Determinants and predictivity.* (Unpublished doctoral dissertation). Acta Universitatis Tamperensis, Tampere.

Mäntymaa, M., Puura, K., Kaukonen, P., Salmelin, R. K., & Tamminen, T. (2008). Infants' social withdrawal and parents' mental health. *Infant Behavior and Development, 31*, 606–613.

Matthey, S., Crncec, R., & Guedeney, A. A. (DATE). *Description of the modified ADBB (m-ADMBB): An instrument to assess for infant withdrawal.* Unpublished manuscript.

Matthey, S., Guedeney, A., Starakis, N., & Barnett, B. (2005). Assessing the social behavior of infants: Use of the ADBB scale and relationship to mother's mood. *Infant Mental Health Journal, 26*, 442–458.

Milne, L., Greenway, P., & Guedeney, A. (2009). Long term developmental impact of social withdrawal in infants. *Infant Behavior and Development, 32*, 159–166.

Murray, L., Fiori-Cowley, A., Hooper, R., & Cooper, P. (1996). The impact of postnatal depression and associated adversity on early mother–infant interactions and later infant outcome. *Child Development, 67*, 2512–2526.

Murray, L., & Trevarthen, C. (1986). The infant's role in mother–infant communication. *Journal of Child Language, 13*, 15–29.

Pageat, P. (1995). *Pathologie du comportement du chien.* Maisons-Alfort, France: Editions du Point Vétérinaire.

Panksepp, J. (2006). Emotional endophenotypes in evolutionary psychiatry. *Progress in Neuropsychopharmacology Biology and Psychiatry, 30*, 774–784.

Puura, K., Guedeney, A., Mantymaa, M., & Tamminen, T. (2007). Detecting children in need: How complicated measures are necessary? *Infant Mental Health Journal, 28*, 409–421.

Puura, K., Mäntymaa, M., Luoma, I., Kaukonen, P., Guedeney, A., Salmelin, R., et al. (2010). Infants' social withdrawal symptoms assessed with a direct infant observation method in primary health care. *Infant Behavior and Development, 33*(4), 579–588.

Robertson, J., & Bowlby, J. (1952). Responses to young children to separation from their mothers. *Courrier du Centre International de l'Enfance, 2*, 131–142.

Rochette, J., & Mellier, D. (2007). The ADBB scale used in preventive strategies for working in network between baby clinic and child mental health service. *Devenir, 19*, 81–108.

Seligman, M.P.E., Abramson, L. Y., Semmel, A., & von Baeyer, C. (1979). Depressive attributional style. *Journal of Abnormal Psychology, 88*, 242–247.

Sroufe, L. A. (1995). *Emotional development: The organization of emotional life in the early years.* Cambridge: Cambridge University Press.

Teti, D. M., Gelfand, D. M., Messinger, D. S., & Isabella, R. (1995). Maternal depression and the quality of early attachment: An examination of infants, preschoolers, and their mothers. *Developmental Psychology, 31,* 364–376.

Tronick, E. Z., & Weinberg, M. K. (1997). Depressed mothers and infants: Failure to form dyadic states of consciousness. In L. Murray & P. Cooper (Eds.), *Postpartum depression and child development* (pp. 54–84). New York: Guilford Press.

Wendland, J., Gautier, A. C., Wolff, M., Brisson, J., & Adrien, J. L. (2010). Social withdrawal behavior and early signs of autism: A preliminary study using family videos. *Devenir, 22*(1), 51–72.

Winnicott, D. W. (1941). Observation of infants in a set situation. *International Journal of Psychoanalysis, 22,* 229–249.

Zero to Three. (2005). *DC 0-3 R: Diagnostic classification of mental health and developmental disorders of infancy and early childhood* (Rev. ed.). Washington, DC: Author.

APPENDIX

ALARM DISTRESS BABY SCALE (ADBB) 2009 (GUEDENEY)

Each item is rated on a scale from 0 to 4:

    0: No unusual behavior
    1: Slightly unusual behavior
    2: Mild unusual behavior
    3: Clear unusual behavior
    4: Severe unusual behavior

This scale is best rated by the observer on the basis of his or her observations, immediately following the clinical interview. Initially, spontaneous behavior is assessed, then follows stimulation (smile, voice, gesture, touch, etc.) and the evolution along time. The rating is what seems more significant during the whole examination procedure. In case of doubt between two ratings, return to the preceding definition. *In case of doubt, use the lowest rating (0).*

1. FACIAL EXPRESSION: Observer assesses any reduction of facial expressiveness:

    0: Face is spontaneously mobile, expressive, animated
    1: Face is mobile, expressive, but limited in range
    2: Little spontaneous facial mobility
    3: Face is fixed, sad
    4: Face is fixed, frozen, absent

2. EYE CONTACT: Observer assesses the reduction of eye contact:

0: Eye contact is spontaneous, easy, and sustained
1: Brief spontaneous eye contact
2: Eye contact is possible only when initiated by observer
3: Eye contact is fleeting, vague, elusive
4: Total avoidance of eye contact

3. GENERAL LEVEL OF ACTIVITY: Observer assesses any failure of motion of the head, torso, and limb without taking into account hand and finger activity:

0: Frequent and well coordinated, spontaneous head, torso, and limb motions
1: Reduced general level of activity, few head and limb movements
2: No spontaneous activity but reasonable level in response to stimulation
3: Very low level of activity in response to stimulation
4: Immobile, rigid, stiff, whatever the stimulation

4. SELF-STIMULATING GESTURES: Observer assesses the frequency with which the child is engrossed with his or her own body activity: fingers, hand, hair, thumb sucking, repetitive rubbing, and so on, in a sort of mechanical, nonpleasurable way that seems detached from the rest of the activity:

0: Absence of self-stimulation; autoexploration is appropriate to the level of general activity
1: Self-stimulation occurs fleetingly
2: Self-stimulation is rare but obvious
3: Frequent self-stimulation
4: Constant self-stimulation

5. VOCALIZATIONS: Observer assesses the lack of vocalization expressing pleasure (cooing, laughing, babbling, babbling with consonant sounds, squealing with pleasure) but also lack of vocalization expressing displeasure or pain (screaming or crying):

0: Frequent, cheerful, modulated spontaneous vocalizations; brief crying or screaming in response to an unpleasant stimulation or sensation
1: Brief spontaneous vocalizations
2: Rare spontaneous vocalizations
3: Whimpering only in response to stimulation
4: Absence of vocalization, even with nociceptive stimulation

6. BRISKNESS OF RESPONSE TO STIMULATION: Observer assesses the sluggishness of response to pleasant or unpleasant stimulation during the examination (smile, voice, touch). The amount of response is

not being assessed here but only the delay in response; *an absence of identifiable response does not allow a rating*:

0: Appropriate, brisk, and swift response to stimulation
1: Slightly delayed and sluggish response to stimulation
2: Sluggish, delayed response to stimulation
3: Markedly sluggish response to even unpleasant stimulation
4: Very delayed response to stimulation or absence of any response to stimulation

7. RELATIONSHIP: Observer assesses the infant's ability to engage in a relationship with him or her or with anyone present in the room other than his or her caretaker. Relationship is assessed through attitude, visual contact, and reaction to stimulation:

0: Relationship clearly and quickly established, rather positive (after a possible initial phase of anxiety) and sustained
1: Relationship identifiable, positive or negative, but less sustained
2: Relationship mildly evident, delayed, positive or negative
3: Doubt as to the existence of a relationship
4: Absence of identifiable relationship to others

8. ATTRACTION: The effort needed by the observer to keep in touch with the child is assessed here, along with the pleasure initiated by the contact with the child *and the subjective feeling of length of time during the examination*:

0: The child attracts attention through his or her initiative and contact, generating a feeling of interest and enjoyment
1: There is interest toward the child, but without less pleasure than as described in 0
2: Neutral feelings toward the child, possibly with a tendency to forget to focus on the child
3: Uneasy feeling toward the child, feeling of being maintained at a distance
4: Disturbing feeling with the child, impression of a child beyond reach

LAST NAME: FIRST NAME: TOTAL:
DATE: / / / AGE: / /MONTHS / / DAYS EXAMINER

Chapter 6

MENTALIZATION AND THE ROOTS OF BORDERLINE PERSONALITY DISORDER IN INFANCY

Peter Fonagy, Patrick Luyten, and Lane Strathearn

Mentalization is a form of social cognition. Human evolutionary history included a point where the ability to predict someone else's response and use that prediction to successfully navigate the social exchange acquired substantial survival value (Humphrey, 1988). To predict people's responses requires understanding their mental state at the time, what they know, how they feel, what they immediately aim to do, what their goals and wishes might be as these states will determine their behavior. The awareness that other people have thoughts and feelings that do not necessarily match our own and that can provide an explanation of their actions has been referred to in the literature as having "theory of mind" (ToM) or "mentalizing" skills (Lieberman, 2007; Saxe, Carey, & Kanwisher, 2004). No animal, not even the most intelligent of nonhuman primates, can always reliably discern the difference between the act of a conspecific due to serendipity and one rooted in intention, wish, belief or desire. The capacity to mentalize has also been argued to account for the other major difference between humans and other apes: (1) self-awareness and self-consciousness as a path to simulation bringing with it social emotions such as embarrassment, shame, and guilt; (2) the species-specific striving to be more than a "beast," to live beyond one's body, to aspire to a spirit that transcends physical reality and step beyond one's own existence; and (3) the social origin of the self in the recognition of oneself in the mental state of the other as the root to a sense of selfhood (see Allen, Fonagy, & Bateman, 2008, for a more comprehensive review of the concept).

As we will discuss in detail later, mentalizing involves inferring mental and emotional states from a range of inputs which include language, nonverbal information which complements language (paralinguistic cues), gestures, facial expressions and other nonverbal cues, such as eye gaze direction. These inputs are however integrated with memories held in semantic or autobiographical memory concerning the other person's likely perspective and belief states (Baron-Cohen, Tager-Flusberg, & Cohen, 2000). Historically the litmus test of rudimentary mentalizing ability was the so-called false belief task which required predicting Sally's (searching) behavior when her knowledge of a piece of physical reality (the location of a ball) was based on a false belief since, unbeknownst to Sally, Ann had moved the ball to another physical location. When Sally comes back into the room, where will she look for the ball, in the place where she left it or the place where the child knows the ball to be? Decades of research using this task in hundreds of studies have demonstrated that false belief performance shows a consistent developmental pattern, even across various countries and various task manipulations (e.g., whether the task objects were transformed in order to deceive the protagonist or not) (Wellman, Cross, & Watson, 2001).

Considering mentalization as meaningfully captured by a simple experimental task does no justice to the concept. For example, there are many tasks tapping the same or similar capacities yielding different developmental models. Using less demanding response modes moves the acquisition of theory of mind forward by at least two years (Surian, Caldi, & Sperber, 2007). Other theory of mind tasks, such as the faux pas task, require greater developmental maturity, perhaps because they require an understanding of false belief to be integrated with an understanding of the emotional impact of beliefs (Stone, Baron-Cohen, & Knight, 1998). Identifying a faux pas requires understanding that someone unintentionally said or did something they should not have (e.g., asking someone what they are going to wear to a party only to discover that the person has not been invited) and that this behavior has emotional consequences. Mentalization is a biologically programmed developmental achievement for all human beings, perhaps similar and linked to language (Harris, 2009).

THE ORIGINS OF MENTALIZATION IN EARLY ATTACHMENT RELATIONSHIPS

Orientation to other minds is part of the behavior repertoire of all infants and the developmental pathway is reasonably well charted (Sharp, Fonagy, & Goodyer, 2008). Weeks after birth the baby smiles at humans (social beings) in preference to objects and from under 12 months babies deliberately engage and redirect their caregiver's attention by pointing and vocalizing. From about nine months the baby differentiates goal oriented actions and imitates others only when this is rational in terms of the actions of the model (Gergely, Bekkering, & Kiraly, 2002; Gergely & Csibra, 2005). By 2.5 years children implement complex social tactics—teasing, lying, saving face. Perspective taking emerges gradually over the first 18 months of life. Children manifest increasing flexibility in using social tactics in middle childhood and by 5–6 will tell "white lies" to protect other people's feelings (not just to avoid punishment) and manifest growing understanding of self-conscious emotions (guilt, embarrassment, pride). Relatively young children will take other people's feelings into account in emotional reactions and manifest concepts of fairness and justice (share things equally) (Sutter & Kocher, 2007). Second-order metarepresentation is thought to be acquired by 6 or 7 (Perner & Lang, 1999).

This early development of theory of mind is not entirely consistent with the neuroimaging studies, which have demonstrated that brain regions supposedly critically involved in mental state attribution (e.g., the medial prefrontal cortex and lateral temporoparietal regions) develop both structurally and functionally at least up to the age of 25. It is not surprising therefore that mental state understanding also continues to develop well past adolescence and probably well into young adulthood (Dumontheil, Apperly, & Blakemore, 2009). The development of the capacity to adopt the other's perspective way beyond infancy speaks to the complexity of the mentalizing process. We believe that it is essential to consider this multifacetedness when applying the mentalizing concept to clinical conditions such as borderline personality disorder (BPD).

A rich developmental psychopathology literature has linked mentalization deficit to a range of clinical conditions, particularly neurological disorders, such as autism, schizophrenia and frontotemporal dementia, which have all been characterized by deficits in mentalizing skills that lead to poor interpersonal relationships and compromised quality of life (Snowden et al., 2003). It is unlikely that these different forms of psychological disturbance could all in some way be causally linked to similar mentalization deficits. We evidently need to identify how different components of mentalizing contribute to the vulnerabilities in interpersonal relationships characteristic of each condition and what neural mechanisms underpin these dysfunctional processes (Luyten, Fonagy, Mayes, & Van Houdenhove, submitted manuscript). In this paper we focus on the way the dysfunction of attachment-related mentalization may explain BPD.

QUALITY OF ATTACHMENT AND EARLY MENTALIZATION

Reddy (2008) offers perhaps the most comprehensive account of factors that contribute to the emergence of mentalization. Reddy proposes that the emergence of mentalization is facilitated by a "second person." She suggests that we come to know of other minds only through interacting with them and observing their responses to us and our responses to them. This requires engagement with the person. Reddy reacts against the traditional literature on mentalization which almost exclusively sees its development as an individual rather than as a social process, despite the evident profound social function of mentalization in human behavior. She makes an ironclad case that knowing minds takes place for both infants and for adults through engagement with minds, so that the richer this engagement the richer a person's representation of mental state is likely to be. Thus the starting point for understanding other minds is not isolation and ignorance but attachment relationships. In a similar vein we have argued that evolution had assigned the attachment relationship the task of conveying knowledge about minds to the human infant and that the quality of the relationship with the attachment figure will therefore impact profoundly on the rate of development and the child's competence in mentalizing.

A number of studies have reported associations between the quality of children's primary attachment relationship and the passing of standard ToM tasks somewhat earlier (Fonagy, Redfern, & Charman, 1997; Fonagy & Target, 1997; Raikes & Thompson, 2006; Symons, 2004). For example, the Separation Anxiety Test, a projective test of attachment security, predicted belief-desire reasoning capacity in 3.5- to 6-year-old children, controlling for age, verbal ability and social maturity (Fonagy, Redfern et al., 1997). In this task the child is asked what a character would feel, based on his or her knowledge of the character's belief. Quality of belief-desire reasoning was predicted from attachment security in infancy: 82% of babies classified as secure at 12 months with mother passed the belief-desire reasoning task at 5.5 years (Fonagy, Steele, Steele, & Holder, 1997). 46% of those who had been classified as insecure failed. Infant–father attachment (at 18 months) also predicted the child's performance.

It should be noted that not all studies have found a relationship between attachment classification and theory of mind tasks. The association is somewhat more likely to be observed for emotion understanding than ToM (Oppenheim, Koren-Karie, Etzion-Carasso, & Sagi-Schwartz, 2005). Given the weak and unreliable association between attachment and measures of mentalization it is most unlikely that the pathway connecting the two is a direct one. Secure attachment and mentalization may both be facilitated by aspects of parenting. The strongest evidence for this comes from observations that the inclination of mothers to take a psychological perspective in relation to their own actions or in relation to their child, including maternal "mind-mindedness" and "reflective function" as they interact with or describe their infants, is associated with both secure attachment and mentalization (Fonagy & Target, 1997; Meins et al., 2002; Sharp, Fonagy, & Goodyer, 2006; Slade, 2005). What qualities of parenting appear to facilitate the establishment of robust mentalization? Precocious understanding of false beliefs has been associated with more reflective parenting practices (Ruffman, Perner, & Parkin, 1999), the quality of parental control (Cutting & Dunn, 1999; Vinden, 2001), parental discourse about emotions (Denham, Zoller, & Couchoud, 1994), the depth of parental discussion involving affect (Dunn, Brown, & Beardsall, 1991) and parents' beliefs about parenting (Ruffman et al., 1999; Vinden, 2001). Parenting of this kind is likely to be strongly associated with the child's acquisition of a coherent conceptual apparatus for understanding behavior in mentalistic terms. It is not hard to understand why parents whose disciplinary strategies focus on mental states (e.g., a victim's feelings, or the nonintentional nature of transgressions) should have children who succeed in understanding the importance of mental states better earlier, as this capacity is reflected in ToM tasks (Charman, Ruffman, & Clements, 2002). By contrast, one might well expect power-assertive parenting (including spanking and yelling) to retard the development of the ability to understand false beliefs (Pears & Moses, 2003). However, in line with the transactional model we advocate, we should consider the possibility that less mentalizing children may be more likely to elicit controlling parenting behavior as well as the parent-to-child causation, that more mindful or reflective parenting facilitates both attachment security and the development of mentalization.

Tolerating negative affect could be a shared characteristic of secure attachment and a family environment facilitating mentalizing. For example, familywide talk about negative emotions, often precipitated by the child's own emotions, has been shown to predict later success on tests of emotion understanding (Dunn & Brown, 2001) and reflecting on intense emotion without being overwhelmed is a marker of secure attachment (Sroufe, 1996). The number of references to thoughts and beliefs and the relationship specificity of children's real-life accounts of negative emotions correlate with early ToM acquisition (false belief performance) (Hughes & Dunn, 2002). There are of course many other characteristics of family function that could link a "secure base" with mentalization. Considering these may be of relevance both from the standpoint of prevention and identifying potentially helpful therapeutic attitudes.

Three programs of work, by Elizabeth Meins (Meins, Ferryhough, Fradley, & Tuckey, 2001), David Oppenheim (Oppenheim & Koren-Karie, 2002) and Arietta Slade and their respective groups (Slade, 2005; Slade, Grienenberger, Bernbach, Levy, & Locker, 2005) have sought to link parental mentalization to the development of affect regulation and secure attachment by examining interactional narratives between parents and children (for a more comprehensive account of these and other investigations of the impact of the parent's capacity to treat the child as a psychological agent on emotional development, see review by Sharp & Fonagy, 2008). These studies demonstrate that (1) mentalizing comments to and about the young child increase the chance of secure attachment and (2) nonmentalizing descriptions of the child reduce the frequency of maternal behaviors that might enhance secure attachment. Mothers' inclination to take the psychological perspective of their child, including maternal mind-mindedness and reflective function in interacting with or describing their infants, has been found to predict not only attachment class but also psychological problems and the child's acquisition of a theory of mind (Fonagy, Steele et al., 1997; Sharp, Fonagy, & Goodyer, 2006).

The findings suggest that a mother's secure attachment history permits and enhances her capacity to explore her own mind and promotes a similar enquiring stance toward the mental state of the infant. The stance is one of open, respectful enquiry that makes use of her awareness of her own mental state to understand her infant, but not to a point where her understanding would obscure a genuine awareness of her child as a separate person. The depth of her awareness of the infant in turn reduces the frequency of behaviors that might undermine the infant's natural progression toward evolving their own sense of mental self through the dialectic of their interactions with the mother. The work of Goldberg and colleagues (Goldberg, Benoit, Blokland, & Madigan, 2003) indeed shows that atypical maternal behavior related not only to infant disorganization of attachment but also to unresolved (disorganized) attachment status on the mother's Adult Attachment Interview (AAI). Thus, while secure mother–infant attachment may not directly facilitate the development of mentalization, it is an indicator of an approach the caregiver takes to the child that may have a direct facilitative effect. Perhaps more crucially, secure infant attachment indicates the absence of aspects of parental behavior that might have undermined mentalization. Preliminary evidence that the capacity for change in attachment organization decreases over development underlines the danger that persistent trauma will lead to long-term disorganization of attachment, with attendant poor development of social cognition and substantially raised risks of psychopathology (Kobak, Cassidy, Lyons-Ruth, & Ziv, 2006). However, we are not suggesting that parental mind-mindedness is inevitably helpful for the child's emotional development. Mind-mindedness is likely to be one of those parental attributes that is most adaptive in moderation. While evidence on this issue is still lacking, on the basis of our clinical observations we have proposed that maladaptive aspects of parental mentalizing of a child can be either deficient (concrete and stimulus bound) or excessive or hypermentalizing (necessarily going beyond the data, often quite distorted and sometimes paranoid). In the research considered earlier, the measure of mind-mindedness was confounded with the accuracy in the scoring; low scorers could be either deficient or excessive mentalizers because both would be rated as failing to reflect the child's mental state with what we may refer to as "grounded imagination" (Allen, 2006). However, regardless of the confounding of accuracy and concreteness in assessments of parenting, the literature suggests that it is not attachment per se but correlated features of parenting, particularly an adult mind taking an interest in a child's mental state, which may be critical in the robust establishment of mentalization.

EARLY ATTACHMENT EXPERIENCES, STRESS REGULATION, MENTALIZATION, AND BPD

A rudimentary version of the hypothesis that BPD involves impairments in mentalization was advanced over 20 years ago (Fonagy, 1989) and we have tried to test and develop the mentalization-based approach to BPD and refine its clinical application in the light of empirical observations by others as well as our own work (Allen et al., 2008; Bateman & Fonagy, 2006; Fonagy & Bateman, 2006). This chapter is a further effort at clarification and expansion with special attention to the role of vulnerability created in infancy. Throughout we have consistently maintained that the capacity to understand the actions of others in terms of putative states of mind (thoughts, feelings, wishes, and desires) is a constitutional potential achieved through social development. We have argued that the acquisition of this capacity occurs through the infant's and young child's engagement with others with whom strong emotional relationships exist, and that the quality of social cognitive engagement will be moderated by the quality of these attachment relationships, particularly but not exclusively, early attachments. Secure attachment is likely to index the resources devoted to the child's subjective experience being contingently responded to (mirrored) by a trusted other, and is associated with the rapid and robust development of mentalization provided that these secure attachment figures possess mentalizing abilities. Part of the formative influence of early attachment arises from its link to the quality of affect mirroring, which in turn impacts on the development of emotion regulative processes and self-control (including attention mechanisms and effortful control) as well as the capacity for mentalization. Disruptions of early attachment with or without later trauma can undermine the capacity for mentalization and, linked to this, create substantial disorganization of the self-structure. An individual's ability to mentalize will vary in quality in relation to their level of emotional stress and their interpersonal context. We have suggested that the emergence of mentalization between the second and fifth year of life is normally antedated by immature forms of subjectivity that nevertheless persist and are revealed when mentalization and the associated capacities for affect representation, affect regulation and attentional control become dysfunctional. Such temporary failures of mentalizing in the context of emotionally intense relationship contexts are characteristic of BPD. The inhibition or decoupling of a mentalizing function at these times causes the apparent "reemergence" of modes of thinking about subjective experience that antedate full mentalization. We have also proposed that limitations in the capacity to experience mental states internally creates a constant pressure for externalization of internal states (projective identification) which is one of the consistent features of dynamic descriptions of BPD. This externalization is also propelled by self-disorganization that includes intolerably painful self-states originally internalized in the course of traumatic experiences to assist coping as part of the self-structure (the self-destructive alien self). A therapeutic intervention that focuses on the patient's capacity to mentalize in the context of attachment relationships can be helpful in improving both behavioral and affective aspects of the condition.

In previous papers we have reviewed evidence in support of these contentions (Fonagy & Bateman, 2007, 2008). In essence we have argued that impairments in social cognition, and particularly a lacking or compromised capacity to understand oneself and others in terms of mental states, play an important role in the development of various psychiatric disorders that involve pathology of the self (Sharp et al., 2008), most specifically BPD (Bateman & Fonagy, 2004), antisocial personality disorder (Bateman & Fonagy, 2008b), and eating disorders (Skarderud, 2007b, 2007c). Over the last decades, several prevention and treatment programs for a variety of disorders and problem behaviors have been developed and some have been evaluated in randomized controlled studies (e.g., Bateman & Fonagy, 2008a). We always assumed that mentalization was a dynamic process that was influenced by stress, and attachment stress in particular. In earlier papers we proposed that, at extreme levels, the activation of the attachment system is associated with a deactivation of the mentalization system along with other emotion-induced cognitive dysfunction. The disorganization of the attachment system has been recognized as a key aspect of the psychopathology of BPD (Gunderson & Lyons-Ruth, 2008).

A schematic representation of our proposals is presented in Figure 6.1. We suggest that genetic and early environmental factors may undermine the development of mentalized affectivity (second-order representations of emotional states). The resulting limitations of infant affect regulation will undermine the development of effortful control and the development of a robust understanding of others as motivated by mental states. These are, as with most developmental processes, potentially interactive and bidirectional in terms of causation. Poor affect regulation obviously makes sensitive caregiving more challenging and the impact of some

Figure 6.1
A schematic developmental model for borderline personality disorder

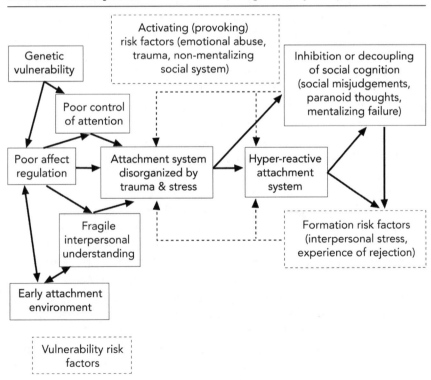

environmental influences are evidently exaggerated by certain genetic attributes (e.g., the short allele of the 5-HTT gene; Barry, Kochanska, & Philibert, 2008). Limitation of voluntarily directing attention and accurate and solid interpersonal understanding contribute to the emergence of a sound behavioral system that underpins mature attachment relationships. We assume that there are several pathways to the development of BPD, depending on the interaction between environmental and biological factors, ranging in severity from individuals that are at increased risk for BPD because of deficits in mentalization (e.g., because they have grown up in a family context characterized by low levels of mentalization and little or no attention to internal mental states), to individuals who are characterized by a defensive decoupling and inhibition of mentalizing because of experiences of abuse and neglect. Moreover, depending on the use of different secondary attachment strategies and contextual factors, some BPD patients will be primarily characterized by preoccupied or avoidant attachment, while in other individuals the attachment system will be disorganized (either from infancy or as a consequence of subsequent stress).

The disorganization of attachment relationships in our view also disorganizes the self-structure, creating incoherence and splitting that makes stress particularly hard to manage. The key consequence of attachment dysregulation in individuals with BPD is the hyperreactivity of the attachment system leading to frantic efforts to avoid abandonment, the diagnostic unstable and intense pattern of interpersonal relationships and a characteristic rapidly escalating tempo moving from acquaintance to great intimacy over extremely brief time periods. We have suggested that the hyperreactivity of the attachment system in these patients, possibly linked with traumatic experiences, may be one of the pathways to impairments of mentalization in BPD—intense affect is incompatible with judgments of social trustworthiness (Fonagy & Bateman, 2008). The vulnerability to an inhibition or decoupling of mentalization may occur for other reasons, such as the understandable reluctance of a maltreated child to contemplate the mental state of adults with frankly destructive thoughts and wishes in relation to her. At these times, mature mentalization gives way in these patients to prementalistic modes of subjectivity whereby the thoughts and feelings lose their as-if quality and become equivalent to physical events, observable physical reality becomes the only criterion for truth and the internal world can genuinely be separated and be experienced as having no real implications for the world outside as in a very extreme form of pretence. Recently accumulated data suggest that a further elaboration of this already complex model may be necessary based on improved understanding to the biology of attachment and the neural basis of mentalization (Luyten et al., 2009).

ATTACHMENT HISTORY AND INDIVIDUAL DIFFERENCES IN STRESS RESPONSIVITY

In the context of secure attachment, the activation of the attachment system predictably involves a relaxation of normal strategies of interpersonal caution. Congruent with this assumption, expressions in most languages associate love with various severe forms of sensory handicap, particularly blindness. There is good evidence that intense activation of the neurobehavioral system underpinning attachment is associated with deactivation of arousal and affect regulation systems (Luyten et al., 2009), as well as deactivation of neurocognitive systems likely to generate interpersonal suspicion—that is, those involved in social cognition or mentalization, including the lateral prefrontal cortex (LPFC), medial prefrontal cortex, lateral parietal cortex, medial parietal cortex, medial temporal lobe, and rostral anterior cingulated cortex (see Fonagy, Luyten, & Strathearn, in press).

The activation and deactivation of the attachment system appears to be closely linked to arousal and stress regulation. Following the model outlined by Mayes (2006) we suggest that with increased arousal there is a switch from cortical to subcortical systems, from controlled to automatic mentalizing and subsequently to nonmentalizing modes. Based on Arnsten's (1998) dual process model, Mayes (2006) proposed that stress regulation is not a generalized state of activation/deactivation but a differential balance of excitation and inhibition involving multiple, interactive neural systems with different neurochemical substrates regulating specific and different aspects of prefrontal, posterior cortical and subcortical functions. For instance, as the level of cortical activation increases through mutually interactive norepinephrine alpha 2 and dopamine D1 systems, prefrontal cortical function improves, including the capacity for attentional control, planning/organization and explicit mentalization. However, with further increases of stimulation, norepinephrine alpha 1 and dopamine D1 inhibitory activity increases to the point that the prefrontal cortex goes "offline" and posterior cortical and subcortical functions (such as more automatic, implicit, affect focused forms of mentalization) are enhanced and finally take over. Increasing levels of norepinephrine and dopamine interact such that above a certain threshold, the balance shifts from prefrontal executive functioning to amygdala-mediated memory encoding and posterior-subcortical automatic responding (fight-flight-freeze).

There are good reasons to suppose that different attachment histories are associated with attachment styles that differ in terms of the associated background level of activation of the attachment system, and the point at which the switch from more prefrontal, controlled to more automatic mentalizing occurs (Luyten et al., submitted manuscript). Dismissing individuals tend to deny attachment needs, asserting autonomy, independence and strength in the face of stress, using attachment deactivation strategies. In contrast, a preoccupied attachment classification or an anxious attachment style are generally thought to be linked with the use of attachment hyperactivating strategies (Cassidy & Berlin, 1994; Mikulincer & Shaver, 2007). Attachment hyperactivating strategies have been consistently associated with the tendency to exaggerate both the presence and seriousness of threats, and frantic efforts to find support and relief, often expressed in demanding, clinging behavior. In the context of this paper, it is important to note that AAI and self-report studies have found a predominance of anxious-preoccupied attachment strategies in BPD patients (Agrawal, Gunderson, Holmes, & Lyons-Ruth, 2004; Fonagy et al., 1996), although there is every indication that the two instruments are sensitive to different forms of psychological dysfunction (Riggs et al., 2007). In one study, 75% of patients meeting criteria for BPD fell into the rarely used subgroup of the AAI (E3): "fearfully preoccupied with respect to trauma" (Fonagy et al., 1996). In borderline patients we and others have noted a characteristic pattern of fearful attachment (attachment anxiety and relational avoidance), painful intolerance of aloneness, hypersensitivity to social environment, expectation of hostility from others, and greatly reduced positive memories of dyadic interactions (e.g., Gunderson & Lyons-Ruth, 2008).

INDIVIDUAL DIFFERENCES IN ATTACHMENT EXPERIENCES AND DEVELOPMENTAL PATHWAYS INVOLVED IN BPD

An important cause of anxious attachment in BPD patients is the commonly observed trauma history of these individuals. Attachment theorists, in particular Mary Main and Erik Hesse, have suggested that maltreatment leads to the disorganization of the child's attachment to the caregiver because of the irresolvable internal conflict created by the need for reassurance from the very person who also (by association perhaps) generates an experience of lack of safety. The activation of the attachment system by the threat of maltreatment is followed by proximity seeking, which drives the child closer to an experience of threat leading to further (hyper)activation of the attachment system (Hesse, 2008). This irresolvable conflict leaves the child with an overwhelming sense of helplessness and hopelessness. Congruent with these assumptions, there is compelling evidence for problematic family conditions in the development of BPD, including physical and sexual abuse (Bandelow et al., 2005; Battle et al.,

2004; Bradley, Jenei, & Westen, 2005), prolonged separations (Soloff & Millward, 1983), and neglect and emotional abuse (Philipsen et al., 2008), although their specificity and etiological import has often been questioned. Probably a quarter of BPD patients have no maltreatment histories and the vast majority of those with abuse histories show a high rate of resilience and no personality pathology (McGloin & Widom, 2001; Paris, 1998).

The familiarity data on BPD is impressive. We know, for instance, that first-degree relatives of a BPD patient could be as much as 10 times more likely to have BPD than the prevalence of BPD in first-degree relatives of schizophrenic patients and explanations in terms of high genetic loading might provide an alternative account for the intrafamilial prevalence of trauma. Nevertheless, findings in support of an etiological role for trauma persist. One study reported a 2.5-fold increase in the risk of BPD for individuals whose mothers suffered a loss within two years of their birth, and a 5.3-fold increase for those with early maltreatment (Liotti & Pasquini, 2000). Maltreatment was implied as a cause in a study of emergent BPD features in school age children (Rogosch & Cicchetti, 2005). In one small longitudinal study, early maltreatment and disrupted parent–infant communication predicted BPD symptoms (Lyons-Ruth, Yellin, Melnick, & Atwood, 2005) and in a larger study verbal (emotional) abuse and neglect even more than physical maltreatment marked out those who went on to develop BPD (Johnson, Cohen, Chen, Kasen, & Brook, 2006). In addition, anomalies in parenting and anxious attachment have been suggested as a possible mediating mechanism between low socioeconomic status and BPD symptoms (Cohen et al., 2008). Early neglect may indeed be an underestimated risk factor, as there is some evidence from adoption and other studies to suggest that early neglect interferes with emotion understanding (e.g., Shipman, Edwards, Brown, Swisher, & Jennings, 2005) and this plays a role in the emergence of emotional difficulties in preschool and even in adolescence. We have suggested that one developmental path to impairments in mentalizing in BPD is a combination of early neglect, which might undermine the infant's developing capacity for affect regulation, with later maltreatment or other environmental circumstances, including adult experience of verbal, emotional, physical and sexual abuse (Zanarini, Frankenburg, Reich, Hennen, & Silk, 2005), that are likely to activate the attachment system chronically (Fonagy & Bateman, 2008). MacDonald and colleagues' (2008) recent observation of elevated posttraumatic stress disorder scores among those 8.5-year-old children exposed to violence who had been disorganized in their attachment with their mothers at 12 months of age is consistent with this suggestion.

We are thus suggesting that BPD symptoms entail an anomaly of co-ordination between frontal and posterior cortical function. There is some evidence for impairments in connectivity of neural systems for orienting to salient input as a key mechanism of the cognitive disturbance and poor impulse control in BPD from MRI studies (Rusch, Luders et al., 2007), EEG studies (e.g., Williams, Sidis, Gordon, & Meares, 2006), studies of brain injury (e.g., da Rocha et al., 2008) and epilepsy (e.g., Tebartz van Elst, 2005). fMRI studies of BPD patients which manipulated the back-ground level of stress and/or attachment system activation (e.g., Minzen-berg, Fan, New, Tang, & Siever, 2007) confirm the abnormal pattern of frontal deactivation and associated hyperresponsiveness of the limbic sys-tem. For example, Silbersweig and colleagues reported that under condi-tions of negative emotion and behavioral inhibition, BPD patients showed relatively decreased ventromedial prefrontal activity (including medial orbitofrontal and subgenual anterior cingulated) and increased amygdalar-ventral striatal activity correlating with decreased constraint (Silbersweig et al., 2007). Findings with implications for the HPA axis function have confirmed that BPD patients, at least those with explicit trauma history, show a reduction in pituitary size (Garner et al., 2007), elevated CSF lev-els of corticotropin-releasing hormone (Lee, Geracioti, Kasckow, & Coc-caro, 2005), dysfunctions of cortisol responsivity (Jogems-Kosterman, de Knijff, Kusters, & van Hoof, 2007), and disturbed dexamethasone sup-pression test response (Wingenfeld et al., 2007). Buchheim and colleagues (2008), for instance, directly challenged the attachment system and ex-amined the functional neuroanatomy of attachment trauma in BPD in a group of 11 female patients and 17 healthy female controls who were told stories in response to seven attachment-related pictures. These researchers found evidence for the hypothesized hyperactivation of the theory of mind system in response to attachment-related stimuli. BPD patients showed significantly more anterior midcingulate cortex activation in response to monadic pictures (characters facing attachment threats alone) and more activation of the right superior temporal sulcus and less activation of the right parahippocampal gyrus in response to dyadic pictures (interaction between characters in an attachment context) compared to controls.

Based on these findings, we propose that a combination of characteris-tics is likely to determine whether an individual "switches" in a particular context from more controlled reflective to automatic mentalization (see Figure 6.1). Anxious-preoccupied attachment strategies, characteristic of many BPD patients, are associated with a lowered threshold for at-tachment system activation and, simultaneously, a lower threshold for controlled mentalization deactivation. Thus, more automatic, subcortical systems, including the amygdala, have a low threshold for responding to stress in BPD patients. This hypothesis in and of itself could offer a comprehensive explanation for one of the central dynamic features of BPD patients, that is, their tendency to form attachments easily and quickly, often resulting in many disappointments. This pattern would be due to their low threshold for activation of the attachment system, and their low threshold for deactivation of neural systems associated with controlled social cognition, including the neural systems involved in judging the trustworthiness of others (Fonagy & Bateman, 2006). The vicious interpersonal cycles that are so characteristic of many BPD patients thus can be understood in terms of excitatory feedback loops leading to increased vigilance for stress-related cues in anxious attachment, particularly attachment characterized by high anxiety and high avoidance. These vicious cycles are also related to their hypervigilance concerning emotional states in others and their failure to distinguish between states of self and others, which further feeds into their lack of self-other differentiation, setting up a likely sequence of further failures in understanding their own internal world, that of others, and the relationship between the two.

In contrast, individuals who use attachment deactivation strategies are able to keep the neural systems involved in controlled mentalization on-line for longer, including neural systems involved in judging the trustworthiness of other individuals (i.e., the "pull mechanism" associated with attachment) (Vrticka et al., 2008). The distinction from securely attached individuals is clear. Secure individuals are able to keep the controlled mentalizing system on-line even in the context of increased stress, which is less likely to trigger the attachment system, while dismissive individuals, for whom mild stress is not likely to trigger the attachment system, may be able to keep mentalization going until the stress becomes severe and the deactivating strategy is likely to fail. If securely attached individuals are those who are able to retain a relatively high activation of prefrontal areas in the presence of the activation of the dopaminergic mesolimbic pathways (attachment and reward system), then differences in mentalization between securely attached and avoidantly/dismissively attached individuals may only show themselves under increasing stress, and this seems concordant with experimental studies.

Although their threshold for switching from controlled to automatic mentalization might be elevated, studies have shown that under increasing levels of stress, these deactivating strategies tend to fail, leading to a strong reactivation of feelings of insecurity, heightened reactivation of negative self-representations, and increased levels of stress (Mikulincer, Gillath, & Shaver, 2002). By contrast, a low threshold for the stress induced activation of the attachment system may translate as easy deactivation of the "pull mechanism" of attachment, and a low threshold for activation of the "push mechanism." In addition, we hypothesize that, if all other factors are constant, the greater an individual's use of hyperactivating strategies, the lower will be their threshold for the activation of automatic mentalization and thus the stronger the relationship between stress and a switch to automatic mentalization will be (Luyten et al., submitted manuscript). Moreover, we predict that greater use of hyperactivating strategies will also be associated with increased time to recovery of mentalization and that deactivating strategies might be associated with relatively rapid recovery of the capacity for mentalization, but these predictions remain to be investigated. However, this model would explain why mentalization deficits in BPD are more likely to be observed in experimental settings that trigger the attachment system, such as in studies collecting AAI narratives (e.g., Fonagy et al., 1996; Levinson & Fonagy, 2004) and also why BPD patients who mix deactivating and hyperactivating strategies, as is characteristic of disorganized attachment, show a tendency for *both* hypermentalization and a failure of mentalization. On the one hand, because attachment deactivating strategies are typically associated with minimizing and avoiding affective contents, BPD patients often have a tendency for hypermentalization, that is, continuing attempts to mentalize, but without integrating cognition and affect. At the same time, because the use of hyperactivating strategies is associated with a decoupling of controlled mentalization, this leads to failures of mentalization as a result of an overreliance on models of social cognition that antedate full mentalizing (Bateman & Fonagy, 2006). Similar conclusions have been drawn from an fMRI study in BPD patients where TAT cards elicited hyperactivation of the anterior cingulate and medial prefrontal cortices, suggesting an overly sensitive switch between emotionally salient and neutral information processing (Schnell, Dietrich, Schnitker, Daumann, & Herpertz, 2007).

Importantly, the switch from controlled to automatic mentalization involves the reemergence of more automatic and often prementalistic modes of thinking about internal states such as the psychic equivalence, the pretend, and the teleological mode of representing the internal world of oneself and others. While psychic equivalence makes subjective experience too real, the pretend mode severs its connection with reality and may even lead to dissociative experiences. The sense of emptiness commonly reported in BPD patients may be an indication of the occasional meaninglessness of subjective experience (Klonsky, 2008). The teleological mode, finally, refers to a mode of thinking that equates thinking about others' desires and feelings with observable behavior. For example, for many patients with BPD, one can only be loved if one is also physically touched.

For many individuals with somatoform disorders, one can only be sick if there is "objective proof" (e.g., medical tests) of one's complaints and sometimes, as in the case of bariatric surgery for obesity in individuals with sexual abuse, professionals respond to such demands teleologically (Morgan, 2008). Evidence for the continued influence on adults of developmentally earlier modes of thought is available from studies of reasoning "errors" (e.g., hindsight bias, "the curse of knowledge," "actions speak louder than words"; Blank, Nestler, von Collani, & Fischer, 2008), which have been used to illuminate the architecture of the belief-desire reasoning processes. The modes of social cognition that are characteristic of the ways of thinking of BPD patients can be understood as prementalistic ways of social reasoning which reemerge with the disappearance of controlled mentalizing. For example, women with BPD not only report higher levels of shame and guilt proneness, they also show greater shame proneness on implicit tests of self-concepts such as the implicit association test (Rusch, Lieb et al., 2007). Shame is felt as "more real" by these patients than anxious patients or normal controls and hence the stronger association with self-esteem and quality of life. The extent to which internal experiences are experienced as if they are real events relates to psychotic features identified in this group, which have been shown to be mediators between histories of childhood sexual abuse and suicidality (Soloff, Feske, & Fabio, 2008). Similar findings are also emerging in relation to anxiety sensitivity in these patients (Gratz, Tull, & Gunderson, 2008).

ATTACHMENT AND RESILIENCE IN BPD

It is well known that individuals with BPD have major problems dealing with adversity. This should hardly surprise us considering that the ability to continue to mentalize even under considerable stress is associated with so-called broaden and build (Fredrickson, 2001) cycles of attachment security, which reinforce feelings of secure attachment, personal agency, and affect regulation ("build"), and lead one to be pulled into different and more adaptive environments ("broaden") (Mikulincer & Shaver, 2007). Congruent with these assumptions, studies on resilience have shown that positive attachment experiences are related to resilience in part through relationship recruiting, that is, the capacity of resilient individuals to become attached to caring others (Hauser, Allen, & Golden, 2006). Hence, high levels of mentalization and the associated use of security-based attachment strategies when faced with stress might explain, at least in part, the effect of relationship recruiting and resilience in the face of stress (Fonagy, Steele, Steele, Higgitt, & Target, 1994). Attachment hyperactivation and deactivation strategies that are typically used by BPD patients, in contrast, can be expected to limit the ability to "broaden and build" in the face of adversity. These strategies have been shown to inhibit behavioral systems that are implicated in resilience, such as exploration, affiliation, and caregiving (Neumann, 2008). These findings may also partially explain BPD patients' difficulties in entering lasting relationships (including relationships with mental health care professionals) and the intergenerational transmission of psychopathology. Hence, when faced with adversity, they have no "security of internal exploration" to find adaptive ways to deal with adversity on their own, nor are they able to effectively recruit others to help them in such situations.

CONCLUSIONS

The mentalization-based approach to BPD aims to provide clinicians with a conceptually sound and empirically supported approach of BPD and its treatment. This chapter presents an extended version of this approach based on recently accumulated data. More specifically, we argue that, although developmentally it is highly likely that different pathways to BPD exist, they all have in common that they result in a low threshold for activation of the attachment system under stress. In combination with low thresholds for deactivation of the capacity for controlled mentalization, particularly with regard to differences in mental states of self versus others, this renders the interpersonal world of individuals with BPD incomprehensible, leading to a cascade of impairments in other aspects of mentalization. This explains BPD patients' propensity to become involved in vicious interpersonal cycles, characterized by marked affective dysregulation. Hence, disruption of the attachment system and identity diffusion closely linked to such disruptions, are seen as the core features of BPD. These are expressed in terms of interpersonal dysfunction and distress and high levels of impulsivity, and result in marked affective dysregulation, as well as feelings of inner pain, shame, and depression. To deal with these feelings, BPD patients rely on a number of maladaptive affect regulation strategies, including self-harm, substance abuse, or hypersexuality. All these involve the reemergence of nonmentalizing modes. These formulations translate into a coherent treatment approach, which may also inform treatment of BPD across various theoretical orientations.

REFERENCES

Agrawal, H. R., Gunderson, J., Holmes, B. M., & Lyons-Ruth, K. (2004). Attachment studies with borderline patients: A review. *Harvard Review of Psychiatry, 12*(2), 94–104.

Allen, J. G. (2006). Mentalizing in practice. In J. G. Allen & P. Fonagy (Eds.), *Handbook of mentalization-based treatment* (pp. 3–30). New York: John Wiley.

Allen, J., Fonagy, P., & Bateman, A. (2008). *Mentalizing in clinical practice.* Washington, DC: American Psychiatric Press.

Arnsten, A.F.T. (1998). The biology of being frazzled. *Science, 280*, 1711–1712.

Bandelow, B., Krause, J., Wedekind, D., Broocks, A., Hajak, G., & Ruther, E. (2005). Early traumatic life events, parental attitudes, family history, and birth risk factors in patients with borderline personality disorder and healthy controls. *Psychiatry Research, 134*(2), 169–179.

Baron-Cohen, S., Tager-Flusberg, H., & Cohen, D. J. (Eds.). (2000). *Understanding other minds: Perspectives from developmental cognitive neuroscience.* New York: Oxford University Press.

Barry, R. A., Kochanska, G., & Philibert, R. A. (2008). G × E interaction in the organization of attachment: Mothers' responsiveness as a moderator of children's genotypes. *Journal of Child Psychology and Psychiatry, 49*(12), 1313–1320.

Bateman, A. W., & Fonagy, P. (2003). Health service utilization costs for borderline personality disorder patients treated with psychoanalytically oriented partial hospitalization versus general psychiatric care. *American Journal of Psychiatry, 160*(1), 169–171.

Bateman, A. W., & Fonagy, P. (2004). *Psychotherapy for borderline personality disorder: Mentalization based treatment.* Oxford: Oxford University Press.

Bateman, A. W., & Fonagy, P. (2006). *Mentalization based treatment for borderline personality disorder: A practical guide.* Oxford: Oxford University Press.

Bateman, A., & Fonagy, P. (2008). 8-year follow-up of patients treated for borderline personality disorder: Mentalization-based treatment versus treatment as usual. *Am J Psychiatry, 165*(5), 631–638.

Battle, C. L., Shea, M. T., Johnson, D. M., Yen, S., Zlotnick, C., Zanarini, M. C., et al. (2004). Childhood maltreatment associated with adult personality disorders: Findings from the Collaborative Longitudinal Personality Disorders Study. *Journal of Personality Disorders, 18*(2), 193–211.

Blank, H., Nestler, S., von Collani, G., & Fischer, V. (2008). How many hindsight biases are there? *Cognition, 106*(3), 1408–1440.

Bradley, R., Jenei, J., & Westen, D. (2005). Etiology of borderline personality disorder: Disentangling the contributions of intercorrelated antecedents. *Journal of Nervous and Mental Disease, 193*(1), 24–31.

Buchheim, A., Erk, S., George, C., Kachele, H., Kircher, T., Martius, P., et al. (2008). Neural correlates of attachment trauma in borderline personality disorder: A functional magnetic resonance imaging study. *Psychiatry Research, 163*(3), 223–235.

Cassidy, J., & Berlin, L. J. (1994). The insecure/ambivalent pattern of attachment: Theory and research. *Child Development, 65*, 971–991.

Charman, T., Ruffman, T., & Clements, W. (2002). Is there a gender difference in false belief development? *Social Development, 11*, 1–10.

Cohen, P., Chen, H., Gordon, K., Johnson, J., Brook, J., & Kasen, S. (2008). Socioeconomic background and the developmental course of schizotypal and borderline personality disorder symptoms. *Development and Psychopathology, 20*(2), 633–650.

Cutting, A. L., & Dunn, J. (1999). Theory of mind, emotion understanding, language, and family background: Individual differences and interrelations. *Child Development, 70*(4), 853–865.

da Rocha, F. F., Malloy-Diniz, L., de Sousa, K. C., Prais, H. A., Correa, H., & Teixeira, A. L. (2008). Borderline personality features possibly related to cingulate and orbitofrontal cortices dysfunction due to schizencephaly. *Clinical Neurology and Neurosurgery, 110*(4), 396–399.

Denham, S. A., Zoller, D., & Couchoud, E. A. (1994). Socialization of preschoolers' emotion understanding. *Developmental Psychology, 30*, 928–936.

Dumontheil, I., Apperly, I. A., & Blakemore, S. J. (2009). Online usage of theory of mind continues to develop in late adolescence. *Developmental Science, 13*(2), 331–338.

Dunn, J., & Brown, J. (2001). Emotion, pragmatics and developments in emotion understanding in the preschool years. In D.B.S. Shanker (Ed.), *Jerome Bruner: Language, culture, self.* Thousand Oaks, CA: Sage.

Dunn, J., Brown, J., & Beardsall, L. (1991). Family talk abut feeling states and children's later understanding of others' emotions. *Developmental Psychology, 27*, 448–455.

Fonagy, P. (1989). On tolerating mental states: Theory of mind in borderline patients. *Bulletin of the Anna Freud Centre, 12*, 91–115.

Fonagy, P., & Bateman, A. W. (2006). Mechanisms of change in mentalization-based treatment of BPD. *Journal of Clinical Psychology, 62*, 411–430.

Fonagy, P., & Bateman, A. (2007). Mentalizing and borderline personality disorder. *Journal of Mental Health, 16*(1), 83–101.

Fonagy, P., & Bateman, A. (2008). The development of borderline personality disorder—a mentalizing model. *Journal of Personality Disorders, 22*(1), 4–21.

Fonagy, P., Leigh, T., Steele, M., Steele, H., Kennedy, R., Mattoon, G., et al. (1996). The relation of attachment status, psychiatric classification, and response to psychotherapy. *Journal of Consulting and Clinical Psychology, 64*, 22–31.

Fonagy, P., Luyten, P., & Strathearn, L. (in press). The roots of borderline personality disorder in infancy: A review of evidence from the standpoint of the mentalization based approach. *Infant Mental Health Journal, 32*, 47–69.

Fonagy, P., Redfern, S., & Charman, T. (1997). The relationship between belief-desire reasoning and a projective measure of attachment security (SAT). *British Journal of Developmental Psychology, 15*, 51–61.

Fonagy, P., Steele, M., Steele, H., Higgitt, A., & Target, M. (1994). The theory and practice of resilience. *Journal of Child Psychology and Psychiatry, 35*, 231–257.

Fonagy, P., Steele, H., Steele, M., & Holder, J. (1997). Attachment and theory of mind: Overlapping constructs? *Association for Child Psychology and Psychiatry Occasional Papers, 14*, 31–40.

Fonagy, P., & Target, M. (1997). Attachment and reflective function: Their role in self-organization. *Development and Psychopathology, 9*, 679–700.

Fredrickson, B. L. (2001). The role of positive emotions in positive psychology: The broaden-and-build theory of positive emotions. *American Psychologist, 56*, 218–226.

Garner, B., Chanen, A. M., Phillips, L., Velakoulis, D., Wood, S. J., Jackson, H. J., et al. (2007). Pituitary volume in teenagers with first-presentation borderline personality disorder. *Psychiatry Research, 156*(3), 257–261.

Gergely, G., Bekkering, H., & Kiraly, I. (2002). Rational imitation in preverbal infants. *Nature, 415*(6873), 755.

Gergely, G., & Csibra, G. (2005). The social construction of the cultural mind: Imitative learning as a mechanism of human pedagogy. *Interaction Studies, 6*, 463–481.

Goldberg, S., Benoit, D., Blokland, K., & Madigan, S. (2003). Atypical maternal behavior, maternal representations, and infant disorganized attachment. *Development and Psychopathology, 15*(2), 239–257.

Gunderson, J. G., & Lyons-Ruth, K. (2008). BPD's interpersonal hypersensitivity phenotype: A gene-environment-developmental model. *Journal of Personality Disorders, 22*(1), 22–41.

Harris, P. L. (2009). Simulation (mostly) rules: A commentary. *British Journal of Developmental Psychology, 27*(Pt. 3), 555–559; author reply 561–557.

Hauser, S. T., Allen, J. P., & Golden, E. (2006). *Out of the woods: Tales of resilient teens.* Cambridge, Mass.: Harvard University Press.

Hesse, E. (2008). The Adult Attachment Interview: Protocol, method of analysis, and empirical studies. In J. Cassidy & P. R. Shaver (Eds.), *Handbook of attachment theory and research* (2nd ed., pp. 552–558). New York: Guilford Press.

Hughes, C., & Dunn, J. (2002). "When I say a naughty word": Children's accounts of anger and sadness in self, mother and friend; Longitudinal findings from ages four to seven. *British Journal of Developmental Psychology, 20*, 515–535.

Humphrey, N. K. (1988). The social function of intellect. In R. W. Byrne & A. Whiten (Eds.), *Machiavellian intelligence: Social expertise and the evolution of intellect in monkeys, apes, and humans* (pp. 13–26). New York: Oxford University Press.

Jogems-Kosterman, B. J., de Knijff, D. W., Kusters, R., & van Hoof, J. J. (2007). Basal cortisol and DHEA levels in women with borderline personality disorder. *Journal of Psychiatric Research, 41*(12), 1019–1026.

Johnson, J. G., Cohen, P., Chen, H., Kasen, S., & Brook, J. S. (2006). Parenting behaviors associated with risk for offspring personality disorder during adulthood. *Archives of General Psychiatry, 63*(5), 579–587.

Klonsky, E. D. (2008). What is emptiness? Clarifying the 7th criterion for border-line personality disorder. *Journal of Personality Disorders, 22*(4), 418–426.

Kobak, R., Cassidy, J., Lyons-Ruth, K., & Ziv, Y. (2006). Attachment, stress and psychopathology: A developmental pathways model. In D. Cicchetti & D. J. Cohen (Eds.), *Development and psychopathology: Vol. 1. Theory and method* (2nd ed., pp. 334–369). New York: John Wiley.

Lee, R., Geracioti, T. D., Jr., Kasckow, J. W., & Coccaro, E. F. (2005). Child-hood trauma and personality disorder: Positive correlation with adult CSF corticotropin-releasing factor concentrations. *American Journal of Psychiatry, 162*(5), 995–997.

Levinson, A., & Fonagy, P. (2004). Offending and attachment: The relationship between interpersonal awareness and offending in a prison population with psychiatric disorder. *Canadian Journal of Psychoanalysis, 12*(2), 225–251.

Lieberman, M. D. (2007). Social cognitive neuroscience: A review of core pro-cesses. *Annual Review of Psychology, 58*, 259–289.

Liotti, G., & Pasquini, P. (2000). Predictive factors for borderline personality dis-order: Patients' early traumatic experiences and losses suffered by the attach-ment figure. The Italian Group for the Study of Dissociation. *Acta Psychiatria Scandanavia, 102*(4), 282–289.

Luyten, P., Mayes, L., Fonagy, P., & Van Houdenhove, B. (2009). *The interper-sonal regulation of stress.* Unpublished manuscript.

Lyons-Ruth, K., Yellin, C., Melnick, S., & Atwood, G. (2005). Expanding the concept of unresolved mental states: Hostile/helpless states of mind on the Adult Attachment Interview are associated with disrupted mother–infant com-munication and infant disorganization. *Development and Psychopathology, 17*(1), 1–23.

MacDonald, H. Z., Beeghly, M., Grant-Knight, W., Augustyn, M., Woods, R. W., Cabral, H., et al. (2008). Longitudinal association between infant disorganized attachment and childhood posttraumatic stress symptoms. *Development and Psychopathology, 20*(2), 493–508.

Mayes, L. C. (2006). Arousal regulation, emotional flexibility, medial amygdala function, and the impact of early experience: Comments on the paper of Lewis et al. *Annals of the New York Academy of Science, 1094*, 178–192.

McGloin, J. M., & Widom, C. S. (2001). Resilience among abused and neglected children grown up. *Dev Psychopathol, 13*(4), 1021–1038.

Meins, E., Ferryhough, C., Fradley, E., & Tuckey, M. (2001). Rethinking mater-nal sensitivity: Mothers' comments on infants mental processes predict secu-rity of attachment at 12 months. *Journal of Child Psychology and Psychiatry, 42*, 637–648.

Meins, E., Fernyhough, C., Wainwright, R., Das Gupta, M., Fradley, E., & Tuckey, M. (2002). Maternal mind-mindedness and attachment security as predictors of theory of mind understanding. *Child Development, 73*, 1715–1726.

Mikulincer, M., Gillath, O., & Shaver, P. R. (2002). Activation of the attachment system in adulthood: Threat-related primes increase the accessibility of mental representations of attachment figures. *Journal of Personality and Social Psychology, 83*(4), 881–895.

Mikulincer, M., & Shaver, P. R. (2007). *Attachment in adulthood: Structure, dynamics and change.* New York: Guilford Press.

Minzenberg, M. J., Fan, J., New, A. S., Tang, C. Y., & Siever, L. J. (2007). Fronto-limbic dysfunction in response to facial emotion in borderline personality disorder: An event-related fMRI study. *Psychiatry Research, 155*(3), 231–243.

Morgan, J. (2008). Binge eating, ADHD, borderline personality disorder, and obesity. *Psychiatry, 7,* 188–190.

Neumann, I. D. (2008). Brain oxytocin: A key regulator of emotional and social behaviours in both females and males. *Journal of Neuroendocrinology, 20*(6), 858–865.

Oppenheim, D., & Koren-Karie, N. (2002). Mothers' insightfulness regarding their children's internal worlds: The capacity underlying secure child–mother relationships. *Infant Mental Health Journal, 23,* 593–605.

Oppenheim, D., Koren-Karie, N., Etzion-Carasso, A., & Sagi-Schwartz, A. (2005, April). *Maternal insightfulness but not infant attachment predicts 4 year olds' theory of mind.* Paper presented at the biennial meeting of the Society for Research in Child Development, Atlanta, GA.

Paris, J. (1998). Does childhood trauma cause personality disorders in adults? *Canadian Journal of Psychiatry, 43*(2), 148–153.

Pears, K. C., & Moses, L. J. (2003). Demographics, parenting, and theory of mind in preschool children. *Social Development, 12,* 1–20.

Perner, J., & Lang, B. (1999). Development of theory of mind and executive control. *Trends in Cognitive Sciences, 3*(9), 337–344.

Philipsen, A., Limberger, M. F., Lieb, K., Feige, B., Kleindienst, N., Ebner-Priemer, U., et al. (2008). Attention-deficit hyperactivity disorder as a potentially aggravating factor in borderline personality disorder. *British Journal of Psychiatry, 192*(2), 118–123.

Raikes, H. A., & Thompson, R. A. (2006). Family emotional climate, attachment security, and young children's emotion knowledge in a high-risk sample. *British Journal of Developmental Psychology, 24*(1), 89–104.

Reddy, V.N.V. (2008). *How infants know minds.* Boston: Harvard University Press.

Riggs, S. A., Paulson, A., Tunnell, E., Sahl, G., Atkison, H., & Ross, C. A. (2007). Attachment, personality, and psychopathology among adult inpatients: Self-reported romantic attachment style versus Adult Attachment Interview states of mind. *Development and Psychopathology, 19*(1), 263–291.

Rogosch, F. A., & Cicchetti, D. (2005). Child maltreatment, attention networks, and potential precursors to borderline personality disorder. *Dev Psychopathol, 17*(4), 1071–1089.

Ruffman, T., Perner, J., & Parkin, L. (1999). How parenting style affects false belief understanding. *Social Development, 8,* 395–411.

Rusch, N., Lieb, K., Gottler, I., Hermann, C., Schramm, E., Richter, H., et al. (2007). Shame and implicit self-concept in women with borderline personality disorder. *Am J Psychiatry, 164*(3), 500–508.

Rusch, N., Luders, E., Lieb, K., Zahn, R., Ebert, D., Thompson, P. M., et al. (2007). Corpus callosum abnormalities in women with borderline personality disorder and comorbid attention-deficit hyperactivity disorder. *Journal of Psychiatry and Neuroscience, 32*(6), 417–422.

Saxe, R., Carey, S., & Kanwisher, N. (2004). Understanding other minds: Linking developmental psychology and functional neuroimaging. *Annual Review of Psychology, 55*, 87–124.

Schnell, K., Dietrich, T., Schnitker, R., Daumann, J., & Herpertz, S. C. (2007). Processing of autobiographical memory retrieval cues in borderline personality disorder. *Journal of Affect Disorders, 97*(1–3), 253–259.

Sharp, C., & Fonagy, P. (2008). The parent's capacity to treat the child as a psychological agent: Constructs, measures and implications for developmental psychopathology. *Social Development, 17*(3), 737–754.

Sharp, C., Fonagy, P., & Goodyer, I. (2006). Imagining your child's mind: Psychosocial adjustment and mothers' ability to predict their children's attributional response styles. *British Journal of Developmental Psychology, 24*(1), 197–214.

Sharp, C., Fonagy, P., & Goodyer, I. (Eds.). (2008). *Social cognition and developmental psychopathology*. Oxford: Oxford University Press.

Shipman, K., Edwards, A., Brown, A., Swisher, L., & Jennings, E. (2005). Managing emotion in a maltreating context: A pilot study examining child neglect. *Child Abuse and Neglect, 29*(9), 1015–1029.

Silbersweig, D., Clarkin, J. F., Goldstein, M., Kernberg, O. F., Tuescher, O., Levy, K. N., et al. (2007). Failure of frontolimbic inhibitory function in the context of negative emotion in borderline personality disorder. *American Journal of Psychiatry, 164*(12), 1832–1841.

Skarderud, F. (2007a). Eating one's words, part I: "Concretised metaphors" and reflective function in anorexia nervosa—an interview study. *European Eating Disorders Review, 15*(3), 163–174.

Skarderud, F. (2007b). Eating one's words, part II: The embodied mind and reflective function in anorexia nervosa—theory. *European Eating Disorders Review, 15*(4), 243–252.

Slade, A. (2005). Parental reflective functioning: An introduction. *Attachment and Human Development, 7*(3), 269–281.

Slade, A., Grienenberger, J., Bernbach, E., Levy, D., & Locker, A. (2005). Maternal reflective functioning, attachment and the transmission gap: A preliminary study. *Attachment and Human Development, 7*(3), 283–298.

Snowden, J. S., Gibbons, Z. C., Blackshaw, A., Doubleday, E., Thompson, J., Craufurd, D., et al. (2003). Social cognition in frontotemporal dementia and Huntington's disease. *Neuropsychologia, 41*(6), 688–701.

Soloff, P. H., Feske, U., & Fabio, A. (2008). Mediators of the relationship between childhood sexual abuse and suicidal behavior in borderline personality disorder. *Journal of Personality Disorders, 22*(3), 221–232.

Soloff, P., & Millward, J. (1983). Developmental histories of borderline patients. *Comprehensive Psychiatry, 24*, 574–588.

Sroufe, L. A. (1996). *Emotional development: The organization of emotional life in the early years.* New York: Cambridge University Press.

Stone, V. E., Baron-Cohen, S., & Knight, R. T. (1998). Frontal lobe contributions to theory of mind. *Journal of Cognitive Neuroscience, 10*(5), 640–656.

Surian, L., Caldi, S., & Sperber, D. (2007). Attribution of beliefs by 13-month-old infants. *Psychological Science, 18*(7), 580–586.

Sutter, M., & Kocher, M. G. (2007). Age and the development of trust and reciprocity. *Games and Economic Behavior, 59*(2), 364–382.

Symons, D. K. (2004). Mental state discourse, theory of mind, and the internalization of self-other understanding. *Developmental Review, 24*, 159–188.

Tebartz van Elst, L. (2005). Towards an integrated model of organic and primary personality disorders. *Z. Epileptologie, 18*, 222–228.

Vinden, P. G. (2001). Parenting attitudes and children's understanding of mind: A comparison of Korean American and Anglo-American families. *Cognitive Development, 16*, 793–809.

Vrticka, P., Andersson, F., Grandjean, D., Sander, D., & Vuilleumier, P. (2008). Individual attachment style modulates human amygdala and striatum activation during social appraisal. *PLoS ONE, 3*, e2868.

Wellman, H. M., Cross, D., & Watson, J. (2001). Meta-analysis of theory-of-mind development: The truth about false belief. *Child Development, 72*(3), 655–684.

Williams, L. M., Sidis, A., Gordon, E., & Meares, R. A. (2006). "Missing links" in borderline personality disorder: Loss of neural synchrony relates to lack of emotion regulation and impulse control. *Journal of Psychiatry and Neuroscience, 31*(3), 181–188.

Wingenfeld, K., Lange, W., Wulff, H., Berea, C., Beblo, T., Saavedra, A. S., et al. (2007). Stability of the dexamethasone suppression test in borderline personality disorder with and without comorbid PTSD: A one-year follow-up study. *Journal of Clinical Psychology, 63*(9), 843–850.

Zanarini, M. C., Frankenburg, F. R., Reich, D. B., Hennen, J., & Silk, K. R. (2005). Adult experiences of abuse reported by borderline patients and Axis II comparison subjects over six years of prospective follow-up. *Journal of Nervous and Mental Disease, 193*(6), 412–416.

Chapter 7

CHILDREN OF PARENTS WITH SUBSTANCE ABUSE AND MENTAL HEALTH PROBLEMS

Vibeke Moe, Torill Siqveland, and Kari Slinning

Substance abuse among parents represents both a prenatal and a postnatal risk to a child's development. Children born to women who have substance abuse problems fall to great risk in terms of developing problems. Substance abuse during pregnancy may affect the child's central nervous system, and the adverse effects of prenatal alcohol exposure are especially well documented. Moreover, consumption of alcohol during pregnancy may lead to fetal alcohol syndrome (FAS) (Streissguth, 1997) or fetal alcohol spectrum disorders (FASD) (Sokol, Delaney-Black, Nordstrom, 2003; Hoyme et al., 2005). Furthermore, children who have been exposed to opioids, such as heroin or methadone during the fetal life, are at risk for suffering from neonatal abstinence syndrome (NAS).

Every year, an unknown number of children are born in Norway with problems that can be traced back to the use of alcohol and drugs by their mothers during pregnancy. Only a miniscule number of these children are identified and receive the particular care and attention that meet their needs. The reasons for this are complex and numerous. Knowledge and experience of how use of drugs and substances impact fetal development are lacking among health care professionals, and substance abuse during pregnancy is still an area that is kept under wraps and faces many taboos, causing it to be an area that is often left largely unexplored by various academics and professionals. Clinicians dealing with these issues often avoid setting a FASD diagnosis for the child in order to avoid stigmatizing mothers who themselves are vulnerable given their often complicated situations. In addition, there is still a lack of evidence-based interventions for these children and their families. Most of the children who are identified live in families where both parents have problems with illegal drug abuse of varying types, and these families also tend to have other problems that could challenge the upbringing of a child. The children of parents who suffer from alcohol abuse are to an even lesser degree identified, as having trouble with alcohol abuse often is a more concealed type of abuse and may occur among families from all kinds of socioeconomic backgrounds.

Even though a proportion of these children end up in foster care or become adopted, an increasing number remain with their biological parents. In Norway there has been a substantial growth in treatment opportunities for pregnant women and families with substance abuse problems the last 10 years. It is important to recognize that substance abuse itself is only one of risk factors for a child's healthy development. For example, we know that these children are more likely to be born prematurely and with low birth weight. Moreover, we know that many of the parents involved suffer from an array of mental health problems, like depression or other types of psychopathology, in addition to their substance abuse problems. Collectively, these factors may negatively impact parents' ability to be sensitive and emotionally available caregivers for their children.

In this chapter we will begin by describing the effects prenatal exposure to substances has on the development of a fetus and the central nervous system of the child, as well as how this reflects on the child later in life through the stages of toddler, small child, and later in childhood. Then we will discuss the importance seeing a child's issues from a background of several combined factors. Although prenatal exposure to drugs and substances is important, factors derived from the child's postnatal care environment also have a significant effect. An awareness of this complexity of factors is a key to tailoring the type of support and treatment many of these families will need. To conclude our work we want to emphasize the vital importance of employing treatment and support models that are comprehensive enough to consider all the aspects involved, including the substance abuse itself, any mental illness issues, parenting roles, self-help skills and last but not least the great need a child has to have caregivers available with the necessary levels of compassion, sensitivity and emotional availability.

THE EFFECTS OF PRENATAL DRUG EXPOSURE TO CHILDREN'S DEVELOPMENT

The brain development of a fetus is vast, and already at birth almost all brain neurons have already been formed. This logically means that the brain is especially vulnerable during pregnancy, and that any exposure to substances in this period may have adverse effects on the development path of the brain. This assumption is supported by, among others, MRI studies that have revealed the organic changes in the brain of children who are exposed to substances prenatal (Walhovd et al., 2007, 2010; Willoughby, Sheard, Nash, & Rovet, 2008).

In addition, there are animal studies that show how prenatal exposure may lead to organic changes in the brain. The advantage of animal studies is that they allow researchers to control for important variables, such as, type of substance, dosage, frequency of exposure, and the time during the pregnancy when the exposure has occurred. When examining children who have been exposed to substances in utero, it is not possible to control for these variables. The results and conclusions can therefore not directly be transferred from animals to humans (Rivkin et al., 2008). When dealing with humans, exposure to substances must always be viewed within a complex framework that includes aspects from genetics, toxicology and nutrition, where possible infections and unknown perinatal circumstances may play a role, not just as a direct effect of the substances (Dixon, 1994; Moe & Slinning, 2002).

People who struggle with substance abuse often consume multiple types of substances including narcotics, medication/psychopharmaca and alcohol. Many of these individuals also have a high consumption of tobacco products, which in and of itself poses a risk factor to the fetus. Smoking during pregnancy can lead to spontaneous abortion, growth problems and premature birth. Even a moderate consumption of cigarettes (5–10 per day) causes the blood circulation in the placenta to be reduced, which leads to a worsened capability of carrying oxygen in the body. Prenatal exposure to nicotine also increases the risk for cot death, and may result in the fall of cognitive functioning in addition to a range of behavioral problems and problems related to attention-deficit hyperactivity disorder (ADHD) (Frank, Augustyn, Knight, Pell, & Zuckerman, 2001; Stene-Larsen, Borge, & Vollrath, 2009).

PRENATAL EXPOSURE TO ALCOHOL

Out of today's most widely known substances, alcohol is the most harmful to a developing fetus. When a pregnant woman consumes alcohol, the fetus reaches the same blood alcohol content (BAC) as the mother, and sustains it for a longer period of time. The alcohol molecule is very small and passes through every cell in the body, with the fetus being no exception. The newly formed cells are especially vulnerable to alcohol, and they may die or change so that they cannot operate optimally. Although the correlation between the amount of alcohol consumed and the sustained effects (dose-response effect) has been well documented, it is true that some fetuses are more susceptible to the harmful effects of alcohol than others, and they can therefore endure lower amounts before neurological effects occur. This is part of the reason why a definite lower limit on alcohol consumption during pregnancy cannot be clearly determined.

FAS is characterized by symptoms that fall into three main categories: pre- and postnatal growth retardation, particular facial features and damage to the central nervous system (CNS). Effects on the CNS may be microcephaly (an undersized brain), hyperactivity, and problems associated with attention deficits. Various degrees of mental retardation is not uncommon. Children with the FAS diagnosis often have problems related to visuomotor skills, and trouble with verbal understanding. Only a fraction of those with severe alcohol-related effects, meet all the criteria to get a FAS diagnosis. Professionals in the field have therefore started using the term FASD instead, as this term more accurately describes the reality that prenatal alcohol exposure may show its effects within a spectrum of symptoms. FASD is an important term as it illustrates how a young child may suffer from exposure to substances even though classical signs might not be apparent, such as the typical facial features. Through spending sufficient time with the child, one will observe how he has trouble adapting to the surroundings and functioning adequately in a variety of situations. The child can have a mood that is unusually volatile depending on the day, he can be very unsettled, more sensitive and react more to changes and deviations in the daily routine or schedule than other young children. Sleep and food intake can differ significantly, and weight problems are common.

The majority of those who are given the FAS diagnosis are children and adolescents in foster care and those who are adopted. The diagnosis is often not given until the children start school when the demands on learning and adequate functioning in society have grown to a new level. At this stage, the problems the child faces are often severe; some can be traced back to the damages by the exposure to substances, while others are secondary or derived problems. This includes issues that develop because the child has not received help early on that is adapted to their needs given their primary problems. Studies done internationally show that children with alcohol-related injuries most often receive the diagnosis, ADHD. This is a limiting diagnosis, since it confines the child from getting all the necessary help it needs within all the areas possibly affected by exposure to alcohol and other substances. Individuals with FASD have more severe cognitive deficits in addition to attention-related, behavioral, social and medical problems. Heart and sight defects are common in this group.

Organic Changes in the Brains of Children Exposed to Alcohol in Utero

Alcohol is defined as a teratogen. This means that alcohol has the potential to cause fetal injuries. Microcephaly is one example. Both human and animal studies have shown that there are several specific areas of the brain that can have reduced size compared to those under normal development. This can apply to the hippocampus, cerebellum, basal ganglia and the frontal lobes. Among other things, the hippocampus is vital for memory and learning. A reduction in the hippocampus has been observed in rats after a single day of fetal alcohol exposure. A central function of the cerebellum is coordination, but it also plays a role in learning and memory. The basal ganglia are involved in both motor and cognitive functions. The frontal lobes are responsible for executive functions in the brain such as the ability to plan, organize, and execute actions. Moreover, a thinner cortex, along with too small or irregularly shaped corpus callosum, has been demonstrated. In addition to these types of structural injuries to the CNS, alcohol during pregnancy can also have an effect on brain cells and reduce both cell division and the creation of new cells. Furthermore, myelination (the process of insulating the nerve cells) can be affected (see Streissguth et al., 2004, for more information on prenatal alcohol exposure and its effects on the CNS).

MRI technology has been used to examine possible connections between symptomatic behavior and organic changes in the brain or injuries. For example, children with FASD often have difficulties with verbal memory, such as recalling what they have learned, and they have difficulties with orienting themselves in space (spatial memory). In one study, children with FASD were compared with children in a control group using cognitive tests and MRIs. Significantly lower total intracranial volume was found in the children with FASD and the hippocampus was especially affected. This was especially true for the left part of the hippocampus (Willoughby et al., 2008).

In another study, children diagnosed with FAS and children who had prenatal alcohol exposure but did not have all of the diagnostic symptoms of FAS were compared with a control group of children. All of the children were examined with an MRI and a battery of neuropsychological tests (Astley et al., 2006). The alcohol-exposed children, regardless of their FAS diagnosis, had significantly higher degrees of neuropsychological problems than the control group. Nevertheless, the children with an FAS diagnosis had the greatest problems out of the three groups. This study also found that the alcohol-exposed groups had significant reduction in total brain volume including the frontal lobes, hippocampus, caudate nucleus, putamen and corpus callosum. The children with an FAS diagnosis had the greatest reduction, but children with FASD also had significantly smaller size of these central parts of the brain than children in the control group.

How Many Children Are Born with Fetal Alcohol Effects in Norway?

International estimates indicate that between 0.5 and 2 of every 1,000 live-born children enter the world with such serious effects of prenatal alcohol exposure that they fill the criteria to be diagnosed with FAS (Astley, Stachowiak, Clarren, & Clausen, 2002; May & Gossage, 2001). Furthermore, it is presumed that at least 3–10 times as many children have alcohol-related effects that cause them to experience difficulties in most areas of daily life. These effects are more difficult to connect with prenatal alcohol exposure because they do not have the classic hallmarks of deformed facial crania (Stratton, Howe, & Battaglia, 1996). Based on international estimates, every year many hundred children in Norway may be born with effects of prenatal alcohol exposure. In light of this, it is interesting to read numbers from the Medical Birth Registry in Norway that show just 17 instances of FAS diagnoses were registered in the period from 1987 to 2005.

NEONATAL ABSTINENCE SYNDROME

Heavy drug abuse, especially where the mothers have used opioids such as heroin or medications like methadone or subutex, often result in serious withdrawal and regulation difficulties in newborn children (Hans & Jeremy, 2001; Lester & Tronick, 1994). Opioids transfer easily through the placenta and have effects on the fetus that are readily observable during the newborn period and can be expressed, among other things, as NAS. Several studies show that children with prenatal opioid exposure to substances like heroin and methadone have lower birth weights and reduced head circumference than children who were not exposed to drugs. Reduced birth weight and head circumference are presumed to be a result of stunted growth during pregnancy and not lower gestational age/being born too early (Hans & Jeremy, 2001). In a Norwegian study of children born to mothers who abused opiates, often combined with other substances, 25% of the children with prenatal drug exposure were born prematurely and had a birth weight under 2,500 grams. The drug exposed children had significantly lower head circumference than children in the control group even after correction was made for prematurity. A large majority of the children suffered from NAS (Moe & Slinning, 2002, 2004).

NAS is defined as a generalized disorder and has a clinical profile with symptoms that include irritability in the CNS and dysfunctions in the autonomic nervous system (ANS), in the esophagus and digestive system and in the respiratory system (Jones, O'Grady, Malfi, & Tuten, 2005; Kaltenbach, Berghella, & Finnegan, 1998). The most commonly used treatment tools for NAS were developed and standardized by Finnegan and colleagues in 1975 and revised for the first time in 1992 (a new revised version is expected sometime in 2010). The form charts to what degree the following symptoms occur: extreme crying, disturbed sleep, hyperactive motor reflexes, shaking/tremors, increased muscle tone, sweating, stuffy nose, sneezing, rapid breathing (respiration rate >60 per minute), regurgitation/severe vomiting, loose bowels, symptoms of failure to thrive and extreme irritability. Treatment depends on how severe the symptoms are, some have many and severe symptoms, while others have few and relatively mild symptoms.

NAS treatment often consists of a combination of pharmaceutical treatment with morphine or opium drops and adaptations in the environment. A central aspect of the abstinence syndrome is hypersensitivity to sound, light and touch. To avoid overstimulation that results in extreme anxiety and irritability in the newborns, the environment needs to be made a sheltered one. Personnel and caregivers also must have necessary knowledge of behavioral conditions and how different conditions guide when it is optimal to achieve contact and enter into interaction with the infant. Another central aspect of the environmentally adapted treatment is to identify and support the infant's emerging self-regulatory abilities.

Methadone-Exposed Infants

Methadone-exposed infants may display more serious NAS symptoms than infants born to mothers who used illegal heroin during pregnancy. Nevertheless, the grades of severity for NAS do not appear to be significantly related to the total dose of methadone taken by the woman during pregnancy (Bakstad, Sarfi, Welle-Strand, & Ravndal, 2009). The reason for this is unknown, but like exposure to other substances, the effect on different fetuses can vary based on various vulnerabilities in different children. It is also important to be aware that due to the long half-life period of methadone, withdrawal symptoms in the child often occur after 48–72 hours (Philipp, Merewood, & O'Brien, 2003). In the United States methadone is recommended as standard treatment for pregnant opiate addicts (National

Institutes of Health Consensus Development Panel, 1998). The main argument for this is that compared with pregnant women who do not receive treatment and who often continue to use illegal substances, it is documented that methadone treatment results in better prenatal care and fetal development along with reduced mortality. The situation in Norway is different from that in the United States. Substitution treatment with medication (methadone or subutex) is given, but there are alternative treatment options for pregnant women with drug abuse problems, especially residential treatment during pregnancy, and this is a preferred treatment form for many pregnant women struggling with drug abuse problems.

How Many Children Are Born with NAS in Norway?

Similar to figures concerning children born with FAS in Norway, we do not have definitive numbers on how many children are born with NAS. There are approximately 40 births among women who have been in substitution treatment annually. These women receive methadone or subutex during pregnancy. It has been demonstrated that around 60% of the children born to these mothers have had withdrawal symptoms that require treatment (Bakstad et al., 2009). We do not have exact figures on the number of births where the fetus has been exposed to illegal opiates and other drugs.

REGULATION DISTURBANCES, COGNITIVE DIFFICULTIES, AND ATTENTION PROBLEMS IN CHILDREN EXPOSED TO OPIATES AND MULTIPLE DRUG USE

The dramatic symptoms that characterize NAS diminish over the course of the first months of life, but it has been noted that even though withdrawal symptoms are a temporary phenomenon, in some cases they may indicate an underlying neurological vulnerability that appears in different ways over the course of development. Among other things, research has shown that many of these children continue to struggle with regulation disturbances and attention problems even after the withdrawal period has ended (Moe & Slinning, 2001; Slinning, 2004).

In the previously mentioned Norwegian study, 136 children were monitored from infancy until they turned 4.5 years old. The children were examined again at 9 and 10–11 years of age. Seventy-eight of these 136 children were prenatally exposed to multiple drug use in which heroin was the primary substance, and they had biological mothers who were serious drug abusers under many strains. A large majority of the children had NAS after birth, and many suffered from great regulation difficulties during infancy. Over the course of their first years of life, over 80% of the drug exposed children were placed in foster care or adopted. The children were examined a total of seven times for mental and motor development, psychosocial development and interaction between the caregiver and child until they were 4.5 years old. At all age levels, the results showed that the drug exposed children scored significantly lower than comparison groups in terms of mental and motor development. This was despite most of the children being placed in foster homes that were specifically selected to give vulnerable children customized care (Moe & Slinning, 2001; Slinning & Moe, 2007). Additional findings showed that at 4.5 years of age the drug exposed children also had specific changes in visual-motor and perceptual skills compared with the control group (Moe & Smith, 2003). Statistical analysis showed that these difficulties appear to be connected with a shorter gestation period, the child's ability to process information during the first year of life and the parents' social economic status. Visual-motor and perceptual skills are presumed to have neuropsychological components, and difficulties in these areas may indicate an underlying neurological weakness that cannot be modified to the same degree as language skills through environmental conditions (Moe, 2002). However, there was great variation among the drug exposed children at the individual level, though none fell within the mental retardation spectrum. In this group developmental gains were made during the first three years of life, something which may be connected with having a good caregiving environment. Unfortunately, the same gains were not observed when the children's development was examined at 4.5 and 9 years of age, respectively. As expected, the control group had about the same scores at each point of measurement.

When the children's socioemotional functions were concerned, it was shown that the drug exposed children had more behavioral problems than children in the control group, and that the behavior changed from internalizing problems to externalizing problems with increased age. At two years of age they were more withdrawn and anxious, while at four years of age they had a greater degree of attention and social difficulties. Markedly higher scores for ADHD-related symptoms were also found among children in the risk group than in the control group, and these problems were mostly expressed at preschool. These results may indicate that the drug exposed children had difficulties with self-regulation since they, in contrast to the control group, showed more problematic behavior at preschool than at home. This could mean that they had difficulty adjusting their own behavior in accordance with the demands of the situation, something that requires both cognitive abilities and the ability to regulate behavior, emotions and motivation (Slinning, 2004; Slinning & Moe, 2007).

One very interesting result from this study is that the prenatally drug exposed boys showed a greater vulnerability than girls until four years of age. It was the boys who scored lowest on average at the time of each measurement, while the girls who were drug exposed had an average that did not differ from the control group. It also showed that the boys' families had more frequent contact with the support system.

Organic Brain Changes in Children Exposed to Opiates and Multiple Drug Use

Animal studies have shown changes in the brains of rat offspring after prenatal exposure to opiates (heroin, methadone and morphine). A reduced density of neurons in the cortex has also been observed, at the same time as the nerve cells' creation of dendrites (branches that, among other things, ensure the connection between the different nerve cells in the brain) is significantly less in morphine exposed offspring than in offspring not exposed to morphine. It has been further indicated that both opiates and cocaine effect neurotransmitter systems (especially monoamine and dopamine transmitter systems) which are associated with the central nervous system's regulation of activation (arousal) and attention (Stanwood & Levitt, 2001).

There are very few studies of children who have been prenatally exposed to opiates and a combination of other drugs where examinations of the brain have been combined with examinations of behavior and development. One exception is our own Norwegian study where MRI (magnetic resonance imaging) examinations were conducted when the children were 10–11 years old (Walhovd et al., 2007). Possible group differences in morphometric cerebral characteristics were examined, and the results showed generally less brain volume in the drug exposed group than in the control group. The areas of the pallidum and putamen were especially hard hit. Reduced volume and injuries in these areas are associated with attention difficulties and hyperactivity in other groups of patients. In the drug exposed group of children we also found a connection between high problem scores for attention and social functioning at nine years of age and less thickness in the cerebral cortex in this area at 11 years of age. Possible group differences in myelination in the brain were also examined with the help of a technique called DTI (diffusion tensor imaging). DTI sequences provide a very detailed picture of the brain. Microstructural differences were found in areas of the brain's white matter in the drug exposed children. There can be several reasons for reduction of white matter, but one possible explanation is that prenatal exposure to drugs may have affected myelination, in other words the insulation of the neural connections in the brain (Walhovd et al., 2010).

As previously mentioned, people who struggle with drug abuse problems often use many different substances, including narcotics, medications and alcohol. This was also the case among mothers in the Norwegian study, even though most of them primarily took heroin. One question this raises is what effect this mixture of different drugs has on the child's central nervous system. In one MRI study conducted by Rivkin et al. (2008) prenatal exposure to cocaine, cigarettes and alcohol was found to have made independent contributions to reduced volume in subcortical gray matter (cgm) and other specific areas, including the putamen and pallidum. Another important finding in this study was that the combination of these substances can affect brain volume and have various effects on the brain structures of prenatally exposed children. This may indicate an accumulative effect of the different substances and possible synergetic effects of the different substances. Multiple drug use brings about effects that cannot be attributed to one particular substance, but likely must be considered to be a result of possible synergetic effects of different substances.

THE IMPORTANCE OF THE CAREGIVING ENVIRONMENT

In many studies of drug exposed children researchers have been mostly interested in finding direct teratological or toxic effects of different substances on the child's cognitive, motor, and behavioral development. This is a very important, but difficult project. To achieve a complete understanding of vulnerable children's needs, we must not overlook other mechanisms that can explain the connection between prenatal drug exposure and the children's development over time. This particularly applies to the importance of the children's postnatal caregiving environment.

Over the past decade there has been an increase in treatment options for drug-addicted pregnant women and parents of young children in Norway. Among other things, there are special addiction treatment institutions with particular responsibility for pregnant women and families with small children. Where pregnant women with serious drug problems are concerned, Social Service Law § 6–2a allows for forcible admission of the woman in order to protect the fetus. "It may be decided that a pregnant drug abuser, without her consent, shall be taken to an institution and held there if the abuse is of such a nature as to make it extremely likely that the child will be born with injuries, and if help measures in accordance with § 6–1 are not sufficient" (Søvig, 1999, p. 48). The conditions that must exist for the involuntary admission paragraph to take effect are, among others, that the abuse may result in injury to the fetus, and that there must be a causal connection between the abuse and the injury. Offers of substitution treatment, often with the medications methadone or subutex, have also become available over the course of the past decade. The increase in treatment options means that today these parents have greater opportunity to take care of their own children than was the case in the early 1990s when the Norwegian study that has been referred to previously was started. As was mentioned, 80% of the drug exposed children had their care taken over during their first year of life.

It is however, well documented that having drug abuse problems is often associated with a host of other risk factors that can affect the ability to be parents. These may be centered on poor somatic health and difficult socio-demographic conditions (Lester, Boukydis, & Twomey, 2000). Drug abuse during pregnancy is also often associated with mental health problems among expectant mothers. Amaro, Zuckerman, and Cabral (1989) found that women struggling with drug abuse are more likely to have a personal and transgenerational history of trauma and abuse; they are more likely to be exposed to violence and have experienced more negative incidents in life than women without drug abuse problems (Beeghly & Tronick, 1994). Numerous studies have documented high incidences of anxiety and depression, along with other serious mental illnesses in addition to little social support (Espinosa, Beckwith, Howard, Tyler, & Swanson, 2001; Luthar, Cushing, Merikangas, & Rousanville, 1998; Savonlahti et al., 2005). It is well documented that maternal depression is a risk factor for the development of the child (Murray, Fiori-Cowley, Hooper, & Cooper, 1996). During interaction with their children, depressed mothers show less reciprocity and synchronicity during interaction, and they fluctuate between being disengaged or intrusive. They are less aware of the child's signals, they can be intrusive, and they can attribute negative characteristics to the child. Children of depressed mothers have also been shown to have less adaptive abilities during interaction than other children (Luthar, D'Avanzo, & Hithes, 2003).

In order to understand what influences an infant's course of development, it is therefore appropriate to focus on the accumulation of risk factors in addition to taking the individual child's vulnerability into consideration. It is not usually isolated factors that make a difference in a child's life, but rather the accumulation of several risk factors in each individual family. The reason that individual factors, such as being low income may seem like a risk on their own, is that they are associated with several other underlying factors. For example, being low income often occurs in families with low levels of education and where there is only one caregiver. This can increase the risk for poverty and low ability to pay, something which may then lead to depression, and can influence the ability to be an emotionally available parent over shorter or longer periods of time (Sameroff & Fiese, 2000). A cumulative risk model emphasizes that the total number of risk factors a child is exposed to is critically important for predicting maladaptivity or poor development. It has been pointed out that it might be that some risk factors really stand out, for example, exposure to alcohol and illegal drugs during gestation. Yumoto, Jacobson, Joseph, and Jacobson (2008) studied two groups of children: one drug exposed group and one group that was not exposed to drugs. They found that four or five risk factors constituted the cutoff point for worse cognitive and behavioral development outcomes in the nonexposed group, while the drug exposed group demonstrated greater vulnerability at lower levels of environmental risks.

Looking at statistics of what may explain development over time in a group of children, differences in the individual characteristics of the person or the family will only explain a small portion of the variation in behavioral development. To be able to really understand which factors are meaningful for development, the surroundings that individuals and families live in have to be considered in their entirety. In other words, it is important to look at both the proximate factors (characteristics of the child like temperament and congenital neurological vulnerability, e.g., and the close interaction between the child and the parents) and the more distal factors (e.g., related to the parents' general socioeconomic status). It is well documented that distal risk factors such as poverty, low socioeconomic status and low levels of education among parents can put a child at double risk of a worse developmental outcome (Beeghy & Tronick, 1994). Jeremy and Bernstein (1984) examined a host of risk factors and protective factors that effected mothers' interactions with their infants and found that the total resources a mother had at her disposal predicted the mother's interactive skills better than to what degree she had a drug problem per se (Lester et al., 2000).

TRANSACTION AND INTERACTION

Earlier we pointed out several factors that can constitute a risk that parents with drug problems will struggle with in participating in interaction with their children in a way that is sensitive and promotes development. At the same time, it is important to emphasize that children also have various conditions for entering into interaction with their caregivers, and that drug exposed children may have neurobehavioral dysregulation that make them extra vulnerable to insensitive care.

Central to understanding every child's development is the mutual influence over time that takes place between the child and the social environment the child grows up in. Of course this also applies to children who are neurologically vulnerable, such as children who were exposed to drugs while in utero. The transaction model therefore represents a foundational way of understanding children's development (Sameroff, 2000). Within this understanding, children's development will not be viewed as a result of either the characteristics of the child or their environment alone. On the contrary, development is a product of the continually dynamic interaction between the child and the environmental experiences that the child has in his/her family and its social context over time. Therefore, this model emphasizes the child and the child's environment equally so that experiences in the environment cannot be seen apart from the child (Sameroff & Fiese, 2000).

At the outset, the processes that form the basis of normal development and development of psychopathology are the same, but because of different levels of vulnerability and different environments the development can go in different directions. Where children who have disturbances with a strong neurobiological component are concerned (such as children with FASD), development will be affected both by the child having a difficulty, and by how the interaction transpires over time (transactions through the caregivers interpretation and response, and the influence of the surrounding environment).

Lester and Tronick (1994) have developed a systemic model that is useful for understanding all of the factors that influence the relationship between mothers with drug problems and their children. This systemic model shows the importance of taking into consideration the entire parent–child system and the circumstances around them. The authors emphasize that focusing exclusively on the mother or father as a drug abuser, or solely on the child as drug exposed, does not take into consideration the transaction processes between parent and child in understanding the development of the child over time. The systemic model shows that being a drug abuser is often an indicator of a total lifestyle. This may imply an atypical form of care and interaction that is not very sensitive. This can have a negative effect on a child's development even without drug exposure.

NEED FOR COMPREHENSIVE TREATMENT MODELS: THE PARENTAL ROLE, MENTALIZATION, AND INCREASED SENSITIVITY IN INTERACTION

Both clinical experiences and various studies indicate that interventions aimed solely at the drug problem, or at the drug problem in combination with guidance on parental skills, does not have sufficient effect when one looks at actual interaction between mother and child (Pajulo, Suchman, Kalland, & Mayes, 2006). This is likely due to the treatment not adequately having resulted in increased sensitivity to what the child needs in the interaction. Consequently, to bring about changes that also have a positive effect for the child's development, it is very important that the treatment is focused on the observable interaction between parent and child, and that it contributes to helping parents to become more sensitive to the child's signals and to respond accordingly (Hans, Bernstein, & Henson, 1999). At the same time, it is important to help the mothers increase their capacity for self-regulation, empathy, and tolerance of stress. This way mothers can become better at regulating their children's behavior and feelings. Better conditions for interaction between mother and child occur when mothers receive treatment for depression or other psychological problems (Olson, O'Connor, & Fitzgerald, 2001) and become emotionally available to their children.

In one study of pregnant women and mothers who were in residential treatment with their children at an addiction treatment center, it was found that focusing on the relationship between mother and child was a decisive factor in obtaining a good treatment outcome. It was shown that this resulted in positive outcomes both in relation to remaining drug-free and to mastering the parental role better (Pajulo et al., 2006). Work on the relationship with the child was started during pregnancy by making the mother conscious of the child in her belly through practical preparations such as finding a name for the child and by helping her to envision how the child would turn out. This mentalization work during pregnancy is believed to encourage later interaction between mother and child. In addition, the expectant mother got help to recognize her own ambivalent feelings and to work on her anxiety and depression. After birth the mother received support to reflect about the child's intentions, behavior and feelings and to view these as meaningful. An important part of the treatment was that the therapist contributed to the mothers reflections on the experiences she has had together with the child and to give them meaning. The relationship between the mother and the therapist is supposed to be accepting, and the therapist should accommodate both the mother's positive and negative feelings relating to the child. A very important aspect of supporting the mother's reflective functioning is to help her better understand the child and what the child is expressing and feeling. This way of working, both with the mother's inner representations and her interaction with the child, is aimed at increasing the mother's sensitivity and her reflective functioning or ability to mentalize (Fonagy, 2006; Sadler, Slade, & Mayes, 2006).

Increased sensitivity is an important factor to work on, as mothers with drug problems often have less ability to read the child's signals and a reduced capacity to manage a child who is hard to regulate. They may also feel more easily rejected by the child and have little self-confidence in their role as parents. Many have not experienced caring parents in their own lives, and are therefore dependent on support and help to learn how they can give good care to their own child. Insensitive care is found to be related to disorganized attachment patterns in the child, which in turn is associated with development of internalized difficulties during the ages of preschool and school (Espinosa et al., 2001). To prevent the child from developing an insecure attachment to the caregiver, it is important to work on the dyad between the child and the caregiver regardless of whether the child is living with his/her biological parents, in a foster home or in an adopted family. It can be difficult to obtain good interaction with a child who mainly shows negative affectivity, is difficult to regulate and does not give clear signals. It is therefore key that the parents receive help with how they should respond to the child, be emotionally supportive and stimulate development.

HELP TO SELF-HELP

Another important aspect of treating and rehabilitating drug-addicted parents is training in self-help skills. Many have been on drugs for many years and therefore have not acquired basic knowledge of things like financial management, food preparation, nutrition and cleaning. In recent years there has been more awareness that this is among the key aspects of treatment, and that it is an important prerequisite for being able to manage on one's own later on. More treatment institutions now give their residents responsibility for practical tasks such as common meals. In addition, they are given responsibility for their own apartment in preparation for living on their own after their stay at the institution. They are also given training in things like using online banking, making food, cleaning, and so on.

An important factor in being able to function in society is access to education and later opportunities for employment. Many who struggle with drugs have discontinued their schooling. Getting help and the chance to get an education or a job is important for being able to function in society and also contributes better economic conditions. Through education and employment chances also increase for building new relationships and creating a network that represents resources and support. This is also totally decisive in preventing isolation, something which can lead to depression and a return to drug abuse.

THE IMPORTANCE OF EARLY INTERVENTION AND FOLLOW-UP OF THE CHILD

To advance a positive prognosis for the child, intervention must take place as early as possible, and the family's combined needs must be mapped out and taken care of. Parents/foster parents, preschool staff and teachers must be given knowledge and training on how they can best adjust daily life for the child. Getting a thorough understanding of the child's resources and difficulties is completely decisive for how they are met and understood by the people around them. An example of intuitive parental behavior is to pick up and rock a child who is crying. This can be counterproductive for a drug exposed child who is often very sensitive to touch and easily overstimulated. An anxious and crying child can become further anxious with rocking and talk. What is needed is concrete information about how hypersensitive children will calm down best when packed tightly in a blanket or comforter and be protected from overwhelming stimuli.

As has been shown, children with FASD face a host of difficulties. We know that access to early intervention is a protective factor that improves the long-term developmental prospects for vulnerable children. This is also the case for individuals with FASD and other types of substance exposure (Frank et al., 2002; Streissguth, Barr, Kogan, & Bookstein, 1996). The child's cognitive, motor, and social resources should be mapped out in order to be able to start appropriate help as early as possible. Special pedagogical follow-up will be of central importance when the child starts going to preschool, and will be necessary throughout the entire period of schooling. It is also important to create understanding in the surroundings that the child is struggling even though the injuries in many cases are not very visible. Furthermore, somatic examinations should be a part of the treatment plan for drug exposed children because effects on the senses such as poor vision or hearing may result from prenatal alcohol exposure.

There is still a lack of evidence-based intervention programs for children with FASD (see Chandrasena, Mukherjee, & Turk, 2008). Based on these circumstances, in 2001 the Centers for Disease Control and Prevention in the United States provided financial support to develop interventions that were specially designed for children with FASD and their families. Funding was offered to five different projects with a goal of developing interventions targeted at typical difficulties faced by children with FASD (see Chandrasena et al., 2008). The overarching goals for every type of intervention program was to support positive cognitive development in individuals with FASD, reduce secondary difficulties and improve the lives of families who live with children with FASD. Most of these interventions were however worked out for school age children, and also partially for children of preschool age. Nonetheless, there are clearly common elements from these programs that are useful and can be transferred to interventions for families with infants and toddlers. Among other things, emphasis was placed on the great importance of supporting caregivers of children with FASD. The programs varied some, but many of them had in different ways psychoeducational elements aimed at parents on the one hand and emphasis on interaction treatment to bring forth good social development in the children on the other. Where psychoeducational content was concerned, it was centered around help functions that can be found for parents with children who have a "hidden" handicap like this. At the same time, emphasis was placed on the importance of shaping a caregiving environment for these children which is emotionally close, well-structured, overviewable and stable (Streissguth et al., 2004).

CONCLUSION

Today it is well documented that children who are exposed to alcohol during pregnancy are at risk of developing difficulties, and that this can lead to FASD (Hoyme et al., 2005; Sokol, Delaney-Black, & Nordstrom, 2003). Nonetheless, very few children are identified. There is further documentation that children who are exposed to opiates and other drugs during pregnancy are also at risk for imbalanced development and organic brain changes, even though the neurobehavioral effects do not appear to be as extensive as those in children with alcohol-related birth defects (Slinning & Moe, 2007; Walhovd et al., 2007; Walhovd et al., 2009).

At the same time, there is a continued lack of knowledge among professionals who work with child and youth psychological health in Norway about the effects of alcohol and drugs on the fetal brain and what characterizes children with prenatal substance-related difficulties. This reduces the chances for children and parents who struggle with these kinds of difficulties to get the right diagnosis and help. Evaluations of this group of children are often too narrow in relation to the numerous functional areas that may be affected.

As we have pointed out, there has been an increase in treatment options for pregnant women and parents with small children who are struggling with alcohol and drug problems in Norway. The challenge for support systems lies in developing comprehensive treatment models that meet the child's need for good care and at the same time prepares the parents to live a drug-free life. Furthermore, we know that many of the parents who struggle with alcohol and drug abuse also have psychological difficulties such as depression or another type of psychopathology which may influence their ability to be sensitive caregivers. Alcohol and drug abuse among parents is also a complex and complicated problem that influences both child and parent in many ways. This shows that there is a need for integrated treatment models that focus on the drug abuse, psychological difficulties, the parental role, self-help skills and not least, the child's special need for sensitive and emotionally available caregivers.

In spite of better treatment options for biological parents and children together, we know that some of these children will end up in a foster home or be adopted. Even though foster parents and adoptive parents are often caregivers with many resources, it is important to emphasize that these parents may also have extra need for support as caregivers for vulnerable children with special needs.

REFERENCES

Amaro, H., Zuckerman, B., & Cabral, H. (1989). Drug use among adolescent mothers: Profile of risk. *Pediatrics, 84,* 144–151.

Astley, S., Aylward, E., Brooks, A., Carmichael Olson, H., Coggins, T., Davies, J., et al. (2006). Association between brain structure, chemistry, and function as assessed by MRI, MRS, fMRI and neuropsychological testing among children with fetal alcohol spectrum disorders (FASD). *Alcoholism: Clinical and Experimental Research, 30,* 229A.

Astley, S. J., Stachowiak, J., Clarren, S. K., & Clausen, C. (2002). Application of the fetal alcohol syndrome facial photographic screening tool in a foster care population. *Journal of Pediatrics, 141,* 712–717.

Bakstad, B., Sarfi, M., Welle-Strand, G. K., & Ravndal, E. (2009). Opioid maintenance treatment during pregnancy: Occurrence and severity of neonatal abstinence syndrome. A national prospective study. *European Addiction Research, 15,* 128–34.

Beeghly, M., & Tronick, E. Z. (1994). Effects of prenatal exposure to cocaine in early infancy: Toxic effects on the process of mutual regulation. *Infant Mental Health Journal, 15*, 158–175.

Chandrasena, A. N., Mukherjee, R.A.S., & Turk, J. (2008). Fetal alcohol spectrum disorders: An overview of interventions for affected individuals. *Child and Adolescent Mental Health, 14*, 162–167.

Dixon, S. (1994). Neurological consequences of prenatal stimulant drug exposure. *Infant Mental Health Journal, 15*, 134–145.Espinosa, M., Beckwith, L., Howard, J., Tyler, R., & Swanson, K. (2001). Maternal psychopathology and attachment in toddlers of heavy cocaine-using mothers. *Infant Mental Health Journal, 22*, 316–333.

Fonagy, P. (2006). The mentalization-focused approach to social development. In J. G. Allen & P. Fonagy (Eds.), *Handbook of mentalization-based treatment* (pp. 53–100). West Sussex, UK: John Wiley.

Frank, D. A., Augustyn, M., Knight, W. G., Pell, T., & Zuckerman, B. (2001). Growth, development, and behavior in early childhood following prenatal cocaine exposure: A systematic review. *Journal of the American Medical Association, 285*, 1613–1625.

Frank, D. A., Jacobs, R. R., Beeghly, M., Augustyn, M., Bellinger, D., Cabral, H., et al. (2002). Level of prenatal cocaine exposure and scores on the Bayley Scales of infant development: Modifying effects of caregiver, early intervention, and birth weight. *Pediatrics 110*, 1143–1152.

Hans, S. L., Bernstein, V. J., & Henson, L. G. (1999). The role of psychopathology in the parenting of drug-dependent women. *Development and Psychopathology, 11*, 957–977.

Hans, S. L., & Jeremy, R. J. (2001). Postneonatal mental and motor development of infants exposed in utero to opioid drugs. *Infant Mental Health Journal, 22*, 300–315.

Hoyme, H. E., May, P. A., Kalberg, W. O., Kodituwakku, P., Gossage, J. P., Trujillo, P. M., et al. (2005). A practical clinical approach to diagnosis of fetal alcohol spectrum disorders: Clarification of the 1996 Institute of Medicine criteria. *Pediatrics, 115*, 39–47.

Jeremy, R. J., & Bernstein, V. (1984). Dyads at risk: Methadone-maintained women and their four month-old infants. *Child Development, 55*, 1141–1154.

Jones, H. E., O'Grady, K. E., Malfi, D., & Tuten, M. (2005). Methadone maintenance vs. methadone taper during pregnancy: Maternal and neonatal outcomes. *American Journal on Addictions, 17*, 372–386.

Kaltenbach, K., Berghella, V., & Finnegan, L. (1998). Opioid dependence during pregnancy: Effects and management. *Obstetrics and Gynecology Clinics of North America, 25*, 139–151.

Lester, B. M., Boukydis, C.F.Z., & Twomey, J. E. (2000). Maternal substance abuse and child outcome. In C. H. Zeanah Jr. (Ed.), *Handbook of infant mental health* (2nd ed., pp. 161–175). New York: Guilford Press.

Lester, B., & Tronick, E. Z. (1994). The effects of prenatal cocaine exposure and child outcome. *Infant Mental Health Journal, 15*, 107–120.

Luthar, S. S., Cushing, G., Merikangas, K. R., & Rousanville, B. J. (1998). Multiple jeopardy: Risk and protective factors among addicted mothers' offspring. *Development and Psychopathology, 10*, 117–136.

Luthar, S. S., D'Avanzo, K., & Hithes, S. (2003). Maternal drug abuse versus other psychological disturbances: Risks and resilience among children. In S. S. Luthar (Ed.), *Resilience and vulnerability: Adaptation in the context of childhood adversities* (pp. 105–129). Cambridge: Cambridge University Press.

May, P. A., & Gossage, J. P. (2001). Estimating the prevalence of fetal alcohol syndrome: A summary. *Alcohol Research and Health, 25*, 159–167.

Moe, V. (2002). Foster placed and adopted children exposed in utero to opiates and other substances: Prediction and outcome at 4 1/2 years. *Journal of Developmental and Behavioral Pediatrics, 23*, 330–339.

Moe, V., & Slinning, K. (2001). Children prenatally exposed to substances: Gender-related differences in outcome from infancy to 3 years of age. *Infant Mental Health Journal, 3*, 334–350.

Moe, V., & Slinning, K. (2002). Prenatal drug exposure and the conceptualization of long term effects. *Scandinavian Journal of Psychology, 1*, 41–47.

Moe, V., & Smith, L. (2003). The relation of prenatal substance exposure and infant recognition memory to later cognitive competence. *Infant Behavior and Development, 26*, 87–99.

Murray, L., Fiori-Cowley, A., Hooper, R., & Cooper, P. (1996). The impact of postnatal depression and associated adversity on early mother–infant interactions and later infant outcome. *Child Development, 67*, 2512–2526.

National Institutes of Health Consensus Development Panel. (1998). Effective medical treatment of opiate addiction. *JAMA, 280*, 1936–1943.

Olson, H. C., O'Connor, M. J., & Fitzgerald, H. E. (2001). Lessons learned from the study of the developmental impact of parental alcohol use. *Infant Mental Health Journal, 22*, 271–290.

Pajulo, M., Suchman, N., Kalland, M., & Mayes, L. (2006). Enhancing the effectiveness of residential treatment for substance abusing pregnant and parenting women: Focus on maternal reflective functioning and mother–child relationship. *Infant Mental Health Journal, 27*, 448–465.

Philipp, B. L., Merewood, A., & O'Brien, S. (2003). Methadone and breastfeeding: New horizons. *Pediatrics, 111*, 1429–1430.

Rivkin, M. J., Davis, P. E., Lemaster, J. L., Cabral, H. J., Warfield, S. K., Mulkern, R. V., et al. (2008). Volumetric MRI study of brain in children with intrauterine exposure to cocaine, alcohol, tobacco, and marijuana. *Pediatrics, 121*, 741–750.

Sadler, L. S., Slade, A., & Mayes, L. C. (2006). Minding the baby: A mentalization-based parenting program. In J. G. Allen & P. Fonagy (Eds.), *Handbook of mentalization-based treatment* (pp. 271–288). West Sussex, UK: John Wiley.

Sameroff, A. J. (2000). Ecological perspectives on developmental risk. In J. D. Osofsky & H. E. Fitzgerald (Eds.), *WAIMH handbook of infant mental health: Vol. 4. Infant mental health in groups at risk* (pp. 1–33). New York: John Wiley.

Sameroff, A. J., & Fiese, B. H. (2000). Models of development and developmental risk. In C. H. Zeanah (Ed.), *Handbook of infant mental health* (2nd ed., pp. 3–19). New York: Guilford Press.

Savonlahti, E., Pajulo, M., Ahlqvist, S., Helenius, H., Korvenranta, H., & Tamminen, J. P. (2005). Interactive skills of infants with their high-risk mothers. *Nordic Journal of Psychiatry, 59*, 139–147.

Slinning, K. (2004). Foster placed children prenatally exposed to polysubstances—attention-related problems at ages 2 and 4 1/2. *European Child and Adolescent Psychiatry, 131*, 19–27.

Slinning, K., & Moe, V. (2007). Forskning i klinikk; langtidsoppfølging av spedbarn som har vært eksponert for rusmidler i fosterlivet. Den gode starten, Aline barnevernsenter 1907–2007, *Norges barnevern*. Spesialnummer i anledning av Alines 100 års jubileum, 43–52.

Sokol, R. J., Delaney-Black, V., & Nordstrom, B. (2003). Fetal alcohol spectrum disorder. *Journal of the American Medical Association, 290*, 2996–2999.

Søvig, K. H. (1999). *Tvang overfor gravide rusmiddelmisbrukere— sosialtjenesteloven § 6–2a*. Oslo: Kommuneforlaget.

Stanwood, G. D., & Levitt, P. (2001). The effects of cocaine on the developing nervous system. In C. A. Nelson & M. Luciana (Eds.), *Handbook of developmental cognitive neuroscience* (pp. 519–536). Cambridge, MA: MIT Press.

Stene-Larsen, K., Borge, A.I.H., & Vollrath, M. E. (2009). Maternal smoking in pregnancy and externalizing behavior in 18-month-old children: Results from a population-based prospective study. *Journal of the American Academy of Child and Adolescent Psychiatry, 48*, 283–289.

Stratton, K., Howe, C., & Battaglia, F. (1996). *Foetal alcohol syndrome: Diagnosis, epidemiology, prevention and treatment*. Washington, DC: National Academy Press.

Streissguth, A. (1997). *Fetal alcohol syndrome: A guide for families and communities*. Baltimore: Paul H. Brookes.

Streissguth, A. P., Barr, H. M., Kogan, J., & Bookstein, F. L. (1996). *Understanding the occurrence of secondary disabilities in clients with fetal alcohol syndrome (FAS) and fetal alcohol effects (FAE)*. Seattle: University of Washington School of Medicine, Department of Psychiatry and Behavioral Sciences.

Streissguth, A. P., Bookstein, F. L., Barr, H. M., Sampson, P. D., O'Malley, K., & Young, J. K. (2004). Risk factors for adverse life outcomes in fetal alcohol syndrome and fetal alcohol effects. *Journal of Developmental and Behavioral Pediatrics, 25*, 228–238.

Walhovd, K. B., Moe, V., Slinning, K., Due-Tønnessen, P., Bjørnerud, A., Dale, A. M., et al. (2007). Volumetric cerebral characteristics of children exposed to opiates and other substances in utero. *Neuroimage, 36*, 1331–1344.

Walhovd, K. B., Moe, V., Slinning, K., Siqveland, T., Fjell, A. M., Bjørnebekk, A., & Smith, L. (2009). Effects of prenatal opiate exposure on brain development—a call for attention. *Nature Reviews Neuroscience, 10*, 390.

Walhovd, K. B., Westlye, L. T., Moe, V., Slinning, K., Due-Tønnessen, P., Bjørnerud, A., et al. (2010). White matter characteristics and cognition in prenatally opiate and polysubstance exposed children—a diffusion tensor imaging study. *American Journal of Neuroradiology, 31,* 894-900.Willoughby, K. A., Sheard, E. D., Nash, K., & Rovet, J. (2008). Effects of prenatal alcohol on hippocampal volume, verbal learning, and verbal and spatial recall in late childhood. *Journal of International Neuropsychological Society, 14*, 1022–1033.

Yumoto, C., Jacobson, S. W., Joseph, L., & Jacobson, J. L. (2008). Fetal substance exposure and cumulative environmental risk in an African American cohort. *Child Development*, 79, 1761–1776.

Chapter 8

SLEEP DISTURBANCES AND CHILDREN'S WELL-BEING

E. Juulia Paavonen and Outi Saarenpää-Heikkilä

Even though the fundamental function of sleep still remains to be determined, accumulating evidence shows the negative consequences of inadequate sleep for health and well-being. Although our knowledge is mainly based on adult studies, research on children's sleep disturbances has also been importantly increasing over the last decade and the studies have pointed out both similarities and differences among children vs. adults. This chapter gives an overview on the recent findings pertaining to children's sleeping difficulties and their etiology as well as the significance of adequate sleep in children's well-being.

SLEEP DISTURBANCES IN GENERAL

Sleeping difficulties range from simple and minor behavioral sleep problems to more severe disturbances with a definitive biological background, such as obstructive sleep apnea or narcolepsy, and they occur frequently during the entire childhood. Epidemiological studies have shown that approximately one third of all children suffer from sleeping difficulties, although the reported prevalence rates vary largely across different studies. The varying rates are likely to reflect differences in the measurement instruments (i.e., varying questionnaires or informants have been used), the research methodology (i.e., the measurement is based on interviews, questionnaires, actigraphs, or polysomnographs) and the definitions that have been set for sleeping difficulties (i.e., the cutoff criteria for sleep disturbances, or the severity of the disturbance).

Sleep disturbances are particularly common in children and adolescents with psychiatric or neurological disorders. For example, depression and anxiety often express themselves as sleep disturbances, most typically as insomnia or hypersomnia. Moreover, various neurological conditions, such as attention-deficit/hyperactivity disorder (ADHD), developmental delay, autism, or Asperger syndrome are also associated with a higher risk for sleeping difficulties, typically frequent nocturnal awakenings or behavioral sleep disturbances. In such a case sleeping difficulties are considered secondary and they overlap the other behavioral symptoms of the underlying neuropsychiatric disorders. Yet, sleep disturbances owe potential to worsen the behavioral symptoms and exacerbate the course of the primary disorder, and therefore treatment of sleep disorders is usually indicated regardless of its etiologic background. Improvement in sleep quality often leads to amelioration of the behavioral symptoms and improvement of mood.

SLEEP DISTURBANCES IN INFANCY

The childhood sleep disturbances closely reflect the child's developmental level, and therefore the typically manifesting sleep disturbances are specific for the age group and developmental level.

Newborn babies sleep approximately 16 hours a day. The interindividual variation is, however, large and some individuals may sleep up to 20 hours a day, while others can sleep as little as only 12 hours a day. The practical significance of this large variation is not known, but as sleep requirements vary between individuals, the observed variation in early life may at least in part reflect the inborn need for sleep which is thought to be genetically determined. On the other hand, it may also carry some clinical significance as short sleep duration at the age of two years and onward has been linked with lower cognitive performance at the age of six years (Touchette et al., 2007).

Sleep structure is immature during the first months of life, and the five sleep stages that are defined in adult's EEG (light sleep stages SI-II, deep sleep stage SIII-IV, and REM sleep) have not evolved yet, but already during the last trimester of pregnancy two sleep stages, active sleep and quiet sleep, can be distinguished. According to the new classification by the American Association of Sleep Medicine (AASM), three sleep stages are defined in infancy: light sleep (stages NI-II), deep sleep (stage NIII), and REM sleep (stage R). By the age of six months the five sleep stages gradually differentiate along with the maturation of the central nervous system. One sleep cycle is shorter in infancy than later (60 minutes vs. 90 minutes among older children and adults). Early childhood is characterized by particularly high proportion of REM sleep, which has raised discussion over the role of REM sleep in promotion of the brain development and neurological maturation. The ontogenetic hypothesis of the function of REM sleep suggests that REM sleep would be particularly important for the neuronal maturation during the fetal period as the sensory input that stimulates neuronal activity is minimal in the uterus. While there are also many other more or less supported theories on the function of REM sleep, animal studies show that early REM sleep deprivation is related to poorer neuronal development and plasticity (Shaffery, Sinton, Bissette, Roffwarg, & Marks, 2002).

Sleep periods of the newborn infant are relatively short (two to four hours) and they are distributed evenly throughout the day without clear differences between the day and night. During the first six months, also the circadian rhythms evolve. Sleep-wake rhythms are controlled by the biological clock of the brain in the suprachiasmatic nuclei. Although the fetal suprachiasmatic nuclei show rhythmic activity already during the last trimester of pregnancy, the earliest signs of diurnal sleep-wake rhythms, such as rhythmicity in melatonin and cortisol secretion, start to show up no earlier than the age of two to three months (Rivkees, 2003). Thereafter the longest sleep periods will be centralizing at night and the longest wake periods during the day. Nocturnal awakenings, however, remain common till the age of two years.

The most typical sleep disturbance in early childhood (age less than one year) is the sleep association problem, a condition in which the child is habitually occupied with certain practices at sleep onset and is unable to fall asleep in the absence of this set of circumstances. When the child is unable to fall asleep on his or her own, he or she will awaken the parents at night between the physiologically occurring awakenings between two sleep cycles. These awakenings can be exhaustive for the entire family particularly when the child repetitively wakes up in the middle of night crying and requiring immediate parental soothing. The babies who are early self-soothers (i.e., can fall asleep without parental support), tend to be better sleepers at the age of one to two years than the signalers (i.e., those who cannot fall asleep without parental support). Moreover, nocturnal awakenings and difficulties with circadian rhythms are also common in this age group, but they merely reflect immaturity of the central nervous system, and do not necessarily represent true deviations from normality.

Etiology of Sleep Disturbances in Infancy

The sleep disturbances in infancy reflect a multitude of etiological factors covering biological (i.e., developmental), environmental and genetic factors. The larger tendency for nocturnal awakenings in early childhood reflects mainly biological factors: the shorter length of the sleep cycle (about one hour; awakenings are most likely to occur between the sleep cycles), the higher proportion of REM sleep in younger (vs. older) children (the awakening threshold is lower from REM sleep than it is from deep sleep) as well as the immaturity of the circadian system.

In addition, many inherited factors, such as temperamental traits are related to the vulnerability for sleeping difficulties. Rhythmicity, for instance, is considered an essential temperamental dimension in early childhood. Some infants show a higher tendency toward regular rhythms than other infants. Irregular infants will require more parental support to be able to develop and maintain diurnal rhythms, while infants who have an inborn a tendency to regularity, may be able to develop such a rhythm of their own or with lower amount of parental guidance.

Even though the maturation of sleep-wake rhythm is under rigorous neural control, a vast range of environmental factors can intervene it and give rise to sleep disturbances. For example, some adverse features in parenting, such as inconsistency in child care, and ambivalence toward infants' demands as well as experienced insecurity in parenting are related to higher tendency for nocturnal awakenings (Morrell, 1999), but as the study was cross-sectional, the cause-effect relationship cannot be determined. When the infant is irregular and sleeps poorly, difficulties in parenting are more common and they can further impair maternal self-esteem.

Adverse parenting practices and negative attitudes can also reflect maternal psychiatric illness. For example, maternal anxiety and depression have been linked with infant's sleeping difficulties. Traditionally, maternal depression was thought to impair the child–parent relations, which could also manifest as sleeping difficulties. However, the causal pathways are more complicated than just that, because frequent nocturnal awakenings provoked by infant's crying could also impair maternal mood. Studies with experimental sleep restriction have shown that both chronic lack of sleep as well as experimental fragmentation of sleep can affect mood and bring out depressiveness in healthy adults (Bonnet, 2000). In these lines, infant's sleeping difficulties were found to be associated with maternal depression only when both the mother and the infant suffered from sleeping difficulties (Hiscock & Wake, 2001) and most importantly it has been noted that treatment of infant sleeping difficulties does not only consolidate infants' sleep but also reduces maternal depressiveness (Hiscock, Bayer, Hampton, Ukoumunne, & Wake, 2008), which suggests that infants' midnight awakenings can also directly affect maternal mood. The relationship between maternal depression and infant sleep is thus likely to be bidirectional.

Bedtime practices have also been linked with sleeping difficulties. For example, active physical comforting and parental presence at bedtime increase the risk for nocturnal awakenings (Morrell & Steele, 2003). Infants who were put to crib awake and were able to fall asleep without parental support were more likely to sleep through the night at the age of one to two years than the other infants (Burnham, Goodlin-Jones, Gaylor, & Anders, 2002). However, at the age of one month most infants are nursed to sleep and the proportion of these infants gradually decreases, which means that most infants are with age able to learn how to fall asleep on their own. Less well known is why some infants are not able to learn self-soothing.

The ability to self-sooth might reflect the infant's attachment style because it seems to contribute the persistence of sleeping difficulties (Morrell & Steele, 2003). Not only the infants' attachment style and but maternal attachment style, too, may play a role. For example, insecure maternal attachment style (Morrell & Steele, 2003) increased the risk for sleeping difficulties among infants. This risk might be mediated via parenting practices, as it has been reported that securely attached infants, determined using the Strange Situation test at the age of one year, had mothers who tended to be more consistent, more sensitive, and more responsive during the nighttime than the mothers of insecurely attached infants (Higley & Dozier, 2009).

Somatic factors are one important etiology of sleep disturbances in infancy. Somatic illnesses, like allergies and infections can manifest themselves as crying and difficulties to settle down and a higher tendency toward nocturnal awakenings. Painful sensations (i.e., ear infection, gastroesophageal reflux), itching and breathing difficulties may also interrupt sleep. Sleep-disordered breathing is a rare but important cause for difficulties in sleep continuity in infancy.

SLEEP DISTURBANCES AMONG TODDLERS

Bedtime problems and nocturnal awakenings are the most typical sleep disturbances among toddlers. While bedtime struggles are often accompanied with prolonged sleep onset latencies, actual difficulties with sleep initiation are less common. Night wakings, in turn, mainly reflect the immaturity of the central nervous system and they are usually not deviations from normality. As many as a half of the children may wake up one to two times a night until at least the age of two years.

In this age some children will also start to suffer from parasomnias, such as sleep terrors, sleep talking and sleep walking (Kotagal, 2009). They are partial awakenings from specific sleep stages, most typically from deep sleep. Sleep terrors, for instance, result from difficulties to leave deep sleep between the two sleep cycles; during the event the child is confused and agitated, unable to communicate with the parents and not consciously aware of the surroundings. After the event, which typically lasts few minutes, the child falls back to deep sleep. They are typically occasional, not very severe from the intensity, and they are usually not related to adverse daytime consequences.

Sleep-disordered breathing also occurs frequently in this age group and it typically manifests itself as restless sleep, tossing and turning, and profuse sweating is also a typical for the condition. Consequences to daytime functioning can be considerable and sleep fragmentation can impair both cognitive and psychic well-being.

Etiology of Sleep Disturbances among Toddlers

In this age group, difficulties at bedtime are typically maintained by ineffective parental control and inconsistent routines at bedtime. They can also reflect anxiety and fears at bed time. Difficulties in the child–parent interaction, family conflicts and negative emotions are also common in families with poorly sleeping children.

Environmental stress factors or chronic lack of sleep can also increase risk for sleeping difficulties or parasomnias. In vulnerable individuals, sleep deprivation seems to increase tendency for disorganized sleep states during state transitions: both experimental restriction of sleep and forced arousals in adults with a history of sleep walking lead to exacerbation of the symptom (Pilon, Montplaisir, & Zadra, 2008). Certain sleeping habits are also related to sleep disturbances; in this age group cosleeping in particular is related to nocturnal awakenings and difficulties in settling down. As many as 35% of five- to seven-year-old children still come to their parents beds many nights a week (Smedje, Broman, & Hetta, 1999). However, cosleeping is not necessarily the primary cause for the sleeping difficulty, as it can also reflect parental reaction to the child's sleeping difficulties (Simard, Nielsen, Tremblay, Boivin, & Montplaisir, 2008).

In addition, certain temperamental traits, particularly "difficult temperament" which is characterized by intense and negative emotionality, is linked with sleep disturbances in this age (Owens-Stively et al., 1997). Genetic factors can thus also play a role, even though in this age group they remain poorly characterized.

Interestingly, prenatal factors too, may have an own, albeit minor, role in tendency for sleeping difficulties both in early childhood and even later in adolescence. For example, small birth weight, artificial labor, bleeding during pregnancy, prenatal exposure to unprescribed medication or caffeine were linked with sleeping difficulties at the age four to nine years (Shang, Gau, & Soong, 2006).

Large adenoids and tonsils are the main cause of snoring and sleep-disordered breathing in this age group. Allergic rhinitis is also more common in snoring children.

SLEEP DISTURBANCES IN SCHOOL-AGED CHILDREN

In school age and adolescence, insomnia becomes the most common sleep disorder. Primary insomnia is characterized by chronic difficulties with onset and/or maintenance of sleep. It is a symptom that often reflects stress in daily life or other adverse life conditions, such as irregular sleeping habits, use of stimulants, too little exercise, and so on. It may also be related to various underlying neuropsychiatric conditions, such as depression or anxiety disorders, or other medical conditions, like substance abuse or somatic illness.

Circadian rhythm disorders are the most important diagnostic alternatives for insomnia, delayed sleep phase syndrome being the most common circadian rhythm disorder. It is characterized by a phase delay of the circadian system, which manifests as a tendency to stay up late in the evening due to difficulties to fall asleep early enough in the evening. It leads to chronic lack of sleep, showing up as difficulties in waking up in the morning in accordance with the school schedules, as well as daytime tiredness and other behavioral symptoms of sleep debt.

Even though inadequate sleep often results from sleep disturbances, it can also arise without any sleep disturbances and be a consequence of inadequate bedtimes. This condition is called as behavioral restriction of sleep. It is an important and prevalent source for inadequate sleep in adolescence. As the sleep needs vary across individuals, not all short sleepers suffer from chronic lack of sleep. Recognition of those who need more sleep requires an experiment where the length sleep is extended. If chronic sleep deprivation has been a problem, daytime functioning, feelings and behavior will improve along the improvement in sleep duration or sleep quality.

Certain somatic entities can also cause sleep disturbances. Previously mentioned snoring and sleep-disordered breathing are still occurring in adolescence and another important disorder is narcolepsy which tends to break out in youth. Prominent daytime sleepiness is the main feature of narcolepsy but fragmented sleep is almost as typical. Cataplectic attacks are also considerable problem. Narcolepsy is often misdiagnosed as ADHD or learning disturbance.

Etiology of Sleep Disorders in School-Aged Children

In school age, sleeping difficulties typically reflect environmental risk factors that range from irregular bedtimes and poor bedtime routines to use of caffeinated beverages and stress at school. Excessive playing of computer games and watching TV are also related to sleeping difficulties (Paavonen, Pennonen, Roine, Valkonen, & Lahikainen, 2006). High exposure to electronic media in school age predicted sleeping difficulties even several years later, in early adulthood (Johnson, Cohen, Kasen, First, & Brook, 2004).

Interpersonal difficulties are also typical in adolescents with insomnia and difficulties to fall asleep. Moreover, negative parenting increases risk for lower sleep quality, negative mood, anxiety and sleepiness (Brand, Hatzinger, Beck, & Holsboer-Trachsler, 2009). Even poor parental sleep quality poses a risk for adolescents' sleep disturbances (Boergers, Hart, Owens, Streisand, & Spirito, 2007), although this risk might be mediated via negative parenting practices (Brand, Gerber, Hatzinger, Beck, & Holsboer-Trachsler, 2009).

In addition, various traumatic experiences as well as adverse childhood experiences, such as family conflicts have been linked with sleep disturbances both in school-aged children (Gregory, Caspi, Moffitt, & Poulton, 2006) and even later in adulthood (Bader, Schafer, Schenkel, Nissen, & Schwander, 2007), suggesting that childhood stress may have persistent influence on sleep and its quality. Finally, even in this age group attachment style can be part of the sleep problem. For example, preoccupied attachment style was related to poor sleep quality among adults (Niko Verdecias, Jean-Louis, Zizi, Casimir, & Browne, 2009).

Twin studies have suggested that environmental factors play a larger role in sleeping difficulties than genetic factors, even though they too contributed to the risk (Gregory et al., 2006). Although the genetic factors that predispose to sleeping difficulties are poorly defined in adolescence, circadian preference (eveningness in particular) is one inherited factor that has been linked with various sleep problems among adolescents (Gau et al., 2007).

Interestingly, prenatal factors are related to sleeping difficulties even up till adulthood. For example, very low birth weight has been linked obstructive sleep apnea and snoring both in adolescence and early adulthood (Paavonen et al., 2007). Prematurity could affect the growth of the airways or the neuronal mechanisms that control breathing during sleep. Prematurity is also associated with earlier bedtime (Strang-Karlson et al., 2008) and the morning chronotype, particularly in premature infants with normal birth weight, that is, those without intrauterine growth restriction (Strang-Karlsson et al., 2010). Although it is not known what the underlying mechanism is, one possibility is that insults in early life may affect the later rhythmicity through programming of the fetal suprachiasmatic nucleus or the amplitudes of melatonin secretion. On the other hand, sleep disturbances may not be related to prematurity itself, but they could also indirectly reflect other factors related to prematurity, for example, treatment at the intensive care unit or familial factors, such as child–parent relationship in early childhood.

SUMMARY OF THE ETIOLOGY OF SLEEP DISORDERS

To summarize the previous discussion, sleep quality reflects multifactorial background where the risk and protective factors construct an interactive and dynamic network which has components of genetic, biological, and environmental factors and where the cause-effect pathways are often bidirectional (Figure 8.1). In part, sleep disturbances also indicate risk for

Figure 8.1
A theoretical model of the interplay between sleep and behavioral problems

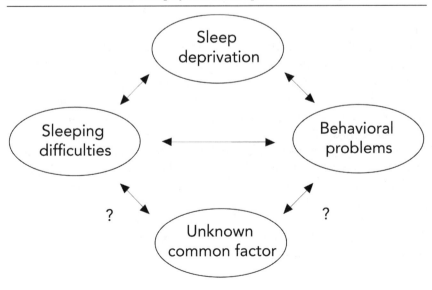

biological vulnerability for neuropsychiatric disorders; it is a nonspecific correlate of the risk, but the interplay of genes and environment, including gene–environment interactions (G × E) and gene–environment correlations (rGE), is also likely to have a role in this complicated relationship. A comprehensive etiological model to explain the risk for sleeping difficulties thus essentially reflects the interplay of environmental and biological factors although the factors that regulate the interplay of environmental and biological factors still remain to be determined.

While the recognition of the risk factors is an important step in understanding causal processes, it is not equivalent to it because the various risk factors can also mirror each other at least to some extent, for example, the effects of parental depression might be mediated via difficulties in parenting and the risks related to cosleeping might reflect the child's inborn difficulties to settle down. Children's sleep quality does not only reflect genetics and the child–parent interaction but environment even more diversely—cultural factors also affect families' sleep practices, parenting and attitudes toward sleep.

WHY IS SLEEP IMPORTANT FOR CHILDREN?

In number of adult studies, short sleep duration and sleeping difficulties, such as insomnia or obstructive sleep apnea, have been linked with negative health outcomes. Poor and short sleep, for example, worsen the glucose tolerance and increase the levels of stress hormones and risk for obesity (Spiegel, Tasali, Leproult, & Van Cauter, 2009) while obstructive sleep apnea has been linked with heart failure and hypertension (Bradley & Floras, 2009).

However, there is a relative lack of studies assessing the significance of adequate sleep among children. For example, the long-term significance of normal sleep-wake rhythm development is poorly characterized, and the significance of the interindividual variability in the sleep structure and its maturation for the neurological and psychological development has not been established.

The consequences of inadequate sleep can be quantitatively in children from those reported among adults, because the need for sleep is larger in early life than later and it can make children particularly vulnerable to the consequences of inadequate sleep. For example, the impact of fragmented sleep was strongest among the youngest children (Sadeh, Gruber, & Raviv, 2002). As sleep is the primary activity of developing brain, an average three-year-old, for instance, has spent more time asleep than in all waking activities, sleep may be even more important for children than it is for adults.

The immaturity of the behavioral compensatory mechanisms can also modify the manifestations of sleep deprivation in children and therefore the consequences of inadequate sleep can be qualitatively different among children as compared to those in adults.

HOW MUCH DO WE NEED SLEEP?

By definition, sleep is sufficient when there is no daytime sleepiness or dysfunction—sleep need is the amount of sleep that guarantees the optimal performance during the next day. Lack of sleep, in turn, leads to negative daytime consequences and impairs performance, functioning and/or well-being one way or another. What the exact consequences of inadequate sleep are may vary between individuals: there seems to be traitlike interindividual variability in the consequences of impaired sleep; different individuals may display different symptom profiles as their re-actions to insufficient sleep. For example, some individuals can be more prone to display tiredness and mood alternations, while others can suffer from deteriorated cognitive performance or inattention when exposed to lack of sleep (Van Dongen, Baynard, Maislin, & Dinges, 2004). In ad-dition, there seems to be persistent differences in the tolerance for lack of sleep at least among adults, so that some individuals seem to be more prone to the negative consequences of inadequate sleep than other indi-viduals (Dinges et al., 1997).

Experimental sleep restriction studies are the best way to study the function of sleep—they will give direct information on the cause-effect relationships. Sleep loss has a well-documented effect on mood and cog-nition among adults. Experimental sleep restriction also impairs perceived psychological well-being and behavior (Banks & Dinges, 2007). Sleep restriction studies among children are limited to those assessing cogni-tive performance and they suggest that the most complex cognitive tasks are being impaired first; restriction of sleep to four hours a night reduced children's performance particularly in tasks requiring verbal creativity and abstract thinking (Randazzo, Muehlbach, Schweitzer, & Walsh, 1998).

Much of our current knowledge about processes beyond sleeping diffi-culties in children comes from epidemiology. Increasing number of cross-sectional studies has linked poor sleep quality or short sleep duration with behavioral problems in healthy children. For example, objectively mea-sured short sleep duration was related to with higher level of behavioral symptoms of ADHD in seven- to eight-year-old children (Paavonen et al., 2009). Poor sleep quality is also related to lower cognitive performance and school performance (Paavonen et al., in press). It may also moderate the cognitive consequences among children risk with other risk factors, such as low educational background (Buckhalt, El-Sheikh, & Keller, 2007) or emotional insecurity or marital conflict in the family (El-Sheikh, Buckhalt, Keller, Cummings, & Acebo, 2007).

Interestingly, short sleep duration in early childhood (under two years of age) is related to poorer cognitive performance at six years of age (Touchette et al., 2007). Early sleeping difficulties may therefore indicate risk for later difficulties, but causal relationship is also possible as one study showed that lengthening of sleep duration improved attention and performance in arithmetic tasks (Sadeh, Gruber, & Raviv, 2003). This suggests that many of the participating children suffered from chronic lack of sleep prior to the study.

During the recent years, there has been discussion over the role of sleeping difficulties in the development of psychiatric disorders. Longitudinal studies have shown that poor sleep quality often predicts depression or other neuropsychiatric disorders. For example, high levels of motor activity during sleep and low regularity in infancy, in particular irregularities in sleeping and eating schedules, were predictive of dysthymic disorder or depression/anxiety in adolescence (Ong, Wickramaratne, Tang, & Weissman, 2006). Similarly, 25% of the children with chronic and severe sleep difficulties at the age of 6–12 months were diagnosed with ADHD at the age of 5.5 years (Thunstrom, 2002). Insomnia or poor sleep quality seem to precede depressiveness in adolescence (Roane & Taylor, 2008) and several studies in adults have also linked poor sleep quality with a higher risk for subsequent depression.

While it is possible that this association reflects a common genetic or neurologic vulnerability for both the psychiatric and the sleep disturbance, the findings have also raised the question, whether sleep disturbances might play a direct and independent causative role in the development of certain psychiatric disorders. Current data, however, does not give definitive answers to this hypothesis as intervention studies are still lacking. If successful treatment of insomnia would decrease the incidence of depression over time, impaired sleep would not only represent a nonspecific correlate of the risk but would be an actual mediator the risk and thereby form an independent risk factor for depression. In accordance with this hypothesis, a recent longitudinal study was able to link earlier bedtimes to lower risk for depression, which suggests that adequate sleep duration could indeed be protective of subsequent depression (Gangwisch et al., 2010).

The connection between sleeping difficulties and ADHD also deserves a specific comment. It has been long known that sleep breathing disorders in children often is accompanied by behavioral symptoms. It was then reported that chronic snoring, a typical symptom of sleep breathing disorder, was more common in children with ADHD than in healthy controls, which that raised question whether a part of the behavioral symptoms of ADHD could be caused by a previously undiagnosed sleep breathing disorder.

There is also clear biological basis for the hypothesis, as the consequences of poor sleep appear to be mediated through the prefrontal cortex which has a central role in regulating executive functions, behavior and alertness (Horne, 1993). A PET-based study, for example, showed that 24 hours of sleep deprivation significantly reduced blood flow in the prefrontal cortex (Thomas et al., 2000) and the degree of this reduced activity corresponded with decreases in those performance tasks that required complex cognitive processing (Belenky et al., 2003). Indeed, one theory suggests that ADHD is a chronic state of hypoarousal where the behavioral symptoms are by-products of the compensatory stimulatory activity of the brain (Cabral, 2006). Clinical observations had already long suggested that children might be prone to displaying behavioral symptoms of ADHD when exposed to lack of sleep (Dahl, 1996). Almost a groundswell of new research was provoked by this fundamental study to explore whether the behavioral symptoms of ADHD and inadequate sleep could be connected.

Studies pertaining to inadequate sleep and the behavioral symptoms in normative populations have been sporadic, but both parent-reported and objectively measured short sleep duration have been linked with behavioral problems, externalizing symptoms, and inattention. Experimental studies have shown that sleep restriction tends to increase inattention but other behavioral aspects, such as impulsivity, have not been covered (Fallone, Acebo, Arnedt, Seifer, & Carskadon, 2001; Fallone, Acebo, Seifer, & Carskadon, 2005). Thus our knowledge on the fundamental role of sleep and the control of behavior, attention, and vigilance still remains elusive.

CONCLUSIONS

Wide range of sleeping difficulties can manifest during the entire childhood. Sleeping difficulties are often persistent and in some cases linked to psychiatric problems at late adolescence, and there is an urgent need to develop and implement prevention programs in the health care system. This would require understanding the patterns of correlation and the dynamic networks between risk factors and their manifestations. Even though inadequate sleep seems to have the potential to impair behavior and performance, intervention studies are needed to confirm the causality. If these studies will confirm the cause-effect relationship, lack of sleep may be an important source of behavioral problems among children, because chronic lack of sleep is a prevalent problem in western societies.

REFERENCES

Bader, K., Schafer, V., Schenkel, M., Nissen, L., & Schwander, J. (2007). Adverse childhood experiences associated with sleep in primary insomnia. *Journal of Sleep Research, 16*(3), 285–296.

Banks, S., & Dinges, D. F. (2007). Behavioral and physiological consequences of sleep restriction. *Journal of Clinical Sleep Medicine, 3*(5), 519–528.

Belenky, G., Wesensten, N. J., Thorne, D. R., Thomas, M. L., Sing, H. C., Redmond, D. P., et al. (2003). Patterns of performance degradation and restoration during sleep restriction and subsequent recovery: A sleep dose-response study. *Journal of Sleep Research, 12*(1), 1–12.

Boergers, J., Hart, C., Owens, J. A., Streisand, R., & Spirito, A. (2007). Child sleep disorders: Associations with parental sleep duration and daytime sleepiness. *Journal of Family Psychology, 21*(1), 88–94.

Bonnet, M. H. (2000). Sleep deprivation. In M. H. Kryger, T. Roth, & W. C. Dement (Eds.), *Principles and practice of sleep medicine* (3rd ed., pp. 53–72). Philadelphia.

Bradley, T. D., & Floras, J. S. (2009). Obstructive sleep apnoea and its cardiovascular consequences. *Lancet, 373*(9657), 82–93.

Brand, S., Gerber, M., Hatzinger, M., Beck, J., & Holsboer-Trachsler, E. (2009). Evidence for similarities between adolescents and parents in sleep patterns. *Sleep Medicine, 10*(10), 1124–1131.

Brand, S., Hatzinger, M., Beck, J., & Holsboer-Trachsler, E. (2009). Perceived parenting styles, personality traits and sleep patterns in adolescents. *Journal of Adolescence, 32*(5), 1189–1207.

Buckhalt, J. A., El-Sheikh, M., & Keller, P. (2007). Children's sleep and cognitive functioning: Race and socioeconomic status as moderators of effects. *Child Development, 78*(1), 213–231.

Burnham, M. M., Goodlin-Jones, B. L., Gaylor, E. E., & Anders, T. F. (2002). Nighttime sleep-wake patterns and self-soothing from birth to one year of age: A longitudinal intervention study. *Journal of Child Psychology and Psychiatry, 43*(6), 713–725.

Cabral, P. (2006). Attention deficit disorders: Are we barking up the wrong tree? *European Journal of Pediatric Neurology, 10*, 66–77.

Dahl, R. E. (1996). The impact of inadequate sleep on children's daytime cognitive function. *Seminars in Pediatric Neurology, 3*(1), 44–50.

Dinges, D. F., Pack, F., Williams, K., Gillen, K. A., Powell, J. W., Ott, G. E., et al. (1997). Cumulative sleepiness, mood disturbance, and psychomotor vigilance performance decrements during a week of sleep restricted to 4–5 hours per night. *Sleep, 20*(4), 267–267.

El-Sheikh, M., Buckhalt, J. A., Keller, P. S., Cummings, E. M., & Acebo, C. (2007). Child emotional insecurity and academic achievement: The role of sleep disruptions. *Journal of Family Psychology, 21*(1), 29–38.

Fallone, G., Acebo, C., Arnedt, J. T., Seifer, R., & Carskadon, M. A. (2001). Effects of acute sleep restriction on behavior, sustained attention, and response inhibition in children. *Perceptual & Motor Skills, 93*(1), 213–229.

Fallone, G., Acebo, C., Seifer, R., & Carskadon, M. A. (2005). Experimental restriction of sleep opportunity in children: Effects on teacher ratings. *Sleep, 28*(12), 1561–1567.

Gangwisch, J. E., Babiss, L. A., Malaspina, D., Turner, J. B., Zammit, G. K., & Posner, K. (2010). Earlier parental set bedtimes as a protective factor against depression and suicidal ideation. *Sleep, 33*(1), 97–106.

Gau, S. S., Shang, C. Y., Merikangas, K. R., Chiu, Y. N., Soong, W. T., & Cheng, A. T. (2007). Association between morningness-eveningness and behavioral/ emotional problems among adolescents. *Journal of Biological Rhythms, 22*(3), 268–274.

Gregory, A. M., Caspi, A., Moffitt, T. E., & Poulton, R. (2006). Family conflict in childhood: A predictor of later insomnia. *Sleep, 29*(8), 1063–1067.

Gregory, A. M., Rijsdijk, F. V., Dahl, R. E., McGuffin, P., & Eley, T. C. (2006). Associations between sleep problems, anxiety, and depression in twins at 8 years of age. *Pediatrics, 118*(3), 1124–1132.

Higley, E., & Dozier, M. (2009). Nighttime maternal responsiveness and infant attachment at one year. *Attachment & Human Development, 11*(4), 347–363.

Hiscock, H., Bayer, J. K., Hampton, A., Ukoumunne, O. C., & Wake, M. (2008). Long-term mother and child mental health effects of a population-based infant sleep intervention: Cluster-randomized, controlled trial. *Pediatrics, 122*(3), e621–627.

Hiscock, H., & Wake, M. (2001). Infant sleep problems and postnatal depression: A community-based study. *Pediatrics, 107*(6), 1317–1322.

Horne, J. A. (1993). Human sleep, sleep loss and behaviour: Implications for the prefrontal cortex and psychiatric disorder. *British Journal of Psychiatry, 162*, 413–419.

Johnson, J. G., Cohen, P., Kasen, S., First, M. B., & Brook, J. S. (2004). Association between television viewing and sleep problems during adolescence and early adulthood. *Archives of Pediatrics & Adolescent Medicine, 158*(6), 562–568.

Kotagal, S. (2009). Parasomnias in childhood. *Sleep Medicine Reviews, 13*(2), 157–168.

Morrell, J. M. (1999). The role of maternal cognitions in infant sleep problems as assessed by a new instrument, the Maternal Cognitions about Infant Sleep Questionnaire. *Journal of Child Psychology and Psychiatry and Allied Disciplines, 40*(2), 247–258.

Morrell, J., & Steele, H. (2003). The role of attachment security, temperament, maternal perception, and care-giving behavior in persistent infant sleeping problems. *Infant Mental Health, 24*(5), 447–468.

Niko Verdecias, R., Jean-Louis, G., Zizi, F., Casimir, G. J., & Browne, R. C. (2009). Attachment styles and sleep measures in a community-based sample of older adults. *Sleep Medicine, 10*(6), 664–667.

Ong, S. H., Wickramaratne, P., Tang, M., & Weissman, M. M. (2006). Early childhood sleep and eating problems as predictors of adolescent and adult mood and anxiety disorders. *Journal of Affective Disorders, 96*(1–2), 1–8.

Owens-Stively, J., Frank, N., Smith, A., Hagino, O., Spirito, A., Arrigan, M., et al. (1997). Child temperament, parenting discipline style, and daytime behavior in childhood sleep disorders. *Journal of Developmental and Behavioral Pediatrics, 18*(5), 314–321.

Paavonen, E. J., Pennonen, M., Roine, M., Valkonen, S., & Lahikainen, A. R. (2006). TV exposure associated with sleep disturbances in 5- to 6-year-old children. *Journal of Sleep Research, 15*(2), 154–161.

Paavonen, E. J., Räikkönen, K., Lahti, J., Komsi, N., Heinonen, K., Pesonen, A. K., et al. (2009). Short sleep duration and behavioral symptoms of attention-deficit/hyperactivity disorder in healthy 7- to 8-year-old children. *Pediatrics, 123*(5), e857–864.

Paavonen, E. J., Räikkönen, K., Pesonen, A.-K., Lahti, J., Komsi, N., Heinonen, K., et al. (in press). Sleep quality and cognitive performance in 8-year-old children. *Sleep Medicine.*

Paavonen, E. J., Strang-Karlsson, S., Räikkönen, K., Heinonen, K., Pesonen, A. K., Hovi, P., et al. (2007). Very low birth weight increases risk for sleep-disordered breathing in young adulthood: The Helsinki Study of very low birth weight adults. *Pediatrics, 120*(4), 778–784.

Pilon, M., Montplaisir, J., & Zadra, A. (2008). Precipitating factors of somnambulism: Impact of sleep deprivation and forced arousals. *Neurology, 70*(24), 2284–2290.

Randazzo, A. C., Muehlbach, M. J., Schweitzer, P. K., & Walsh, J. K. (1998). Cognitive function following acute sleep restriction in children ages 10–14. *Sleep, 21*(8), 861–868.

Rivkees, S. A. (2003). Developing circadian rhythmicity in infants. *Pediatric Endocrinology Review, 1*(1), 38–45.

Roane, B. M., & Taylor, D. J. (2008). Adolescent insomnia as a risk factor for early adult depression and substance abuse. *Sleep, 31*(10), 1351–1356.

Sadeh, A., Gruber, R., & Raviv, A. (2002). Sleep, neurobehavioral functioning, and behavior problems in school-age children. *Child Development, 73*(2), 405–417.

Sadeh, A., Gruber, R., & Raviv, A. (2003). The effects of sleep restriction and extension on school-age children: What a difference an hour makes. *Child Development, 74*(2), 444–455.

Shaffery, J. P., Sinton, C. M., Bissette, G., Roffwarg, H. P., & Marks, G. A. (2002). Rapid eye movement sleep deprivation modifies expression of long-term potentiation in visual cortex of immature rats. *Neuroscience, 110*(3), 431–443.

Shang, C. Y., Gau, S. S., & Soong, W. T. (2006). Association between childhood sleep problems and perinatal factors, parental mental distress and behavioral problems. *Journal of Sleep Research, 15*(1), 63–73.

Simard, V., Nielsen, T. A., Tremblay, R. E., Boivin, M., & Montplaisir, J. Y. (2008). Longitudinal study of preschool sleep disturbance: The predictive role of maladaptive parental behaviors, early sleep problems, and child/mother psychological factors. *Archives of Pediatric & Adolescent Medicine, 162*(4), 360–367.

Smedje, H., Broman, J. E., & Hetta, J. (1999). Parents' reports of disturbed sleep in 5–7-year-old Swedish children. *Acta Paediatrica, 88*(8), 858–865.

Spiegel, K., Tasali, E., Leproult, R., & Van Cauter, E. (2009). Effects of poor and short sleep on glucose metabolism and obesity risk. *Nature Reviews Endocrinology, 5*(5), 253–261.

Thomas, M., Sing, H., Belenky, G., Holcomb, H., Mayberg, H., Dannals, R., et al. (2000). Neural basis of alertness and cognitive performance impairments during sleepiness. I. Effects of 24 h of sleep deprivation on waking human regional brain activity. *Journal of Sleep Research, 9*(4), 335–352.

Thunstrom, M. (2002). Severe sleep problems in infancy associated with subsequent development of attention-deficit/hyperactivity disorder at 5.5 years of age. *Acta Paediatrica, 91*(5), 584–592.

Touchette, E., Petit, D., Seguin, J. R., Boivin, M., Tremblay, R. E., & Montplaisir, J. Y. (2007). Associations between sleep duration patterns and behavioral/cognitive functioning at school entry. *Sleep, 30*(9), 1213–1219.

Van Dongen, H. P., Baynard, M. D., Maislin, G., & Dinges, D. F. (2004). Systematic interindividual differences in neurobehavioral impairment from sleep loss: Evidence of trait-like differential vulnerability. *Sleep, 27*(3), 423–433.

Chapter 9

MENTAL HEALTH OF CHILDREN EVACUATED DURING WORLD WAR II

Anu-Katriina Pesonen and Katri Räikkönen

LONG-TERM CONSEQUENCES OF EARLY LIFE STRESS

Recent research has produced increasing evidence that early life stress (ELS), an experience of severe stress due, for example, to parental loss, abuse, or neglect during the childhood years, may have profound long-term effects on the individual's physiology, psychology, and immune function (Alastalo et al., 2009; Danese et al., 2009; Danese et al., 2008; Gunnar & Quevedo, 2007). This evidence has confirmed observations from experimental animal models in which ELS, usually defined as temporary maternal separation early in life, has shown to cause changes in gene expression that are manifest, for instance, in the physiology of stress regulation (Holmes et al., 2005; Pryce et al., 2005).

However, compared to animal experiments, in which the nature and duration of ELS can be controlled by the experimenter, the examination of ELS in humans is methodologically challenging. Most typically children experience ELS in the form of abuse and neglect in their family environment, and it may be impossible to disentangle the effects of ELS from their shared genetic makeup with their parents. Second, the experience of ELS may be cumulative such that prenatal adversity, economical strains, learning difficulties, nutritional problems, parental mental health problems, lack of appropriate health care, child abuse, and neglect accumulate in a manner that make it impossible to understand which characteristics of ELS may especially be harmful for later mental health. Finally, the major problem in the examination of ELS on later mental health is that most of the studies are conducted on samples in which participants are asked to report their experience of ELS retrospectively. In these studies there is always the possibility that the recall is biased by the current mental health status, or by other life events that have occurred after the childhood years.

With regard to prospective human evidence, adoption studies provide one methodologically sound alternative to study the effects of ELS. Not surprisingly, internationally adopted children have shown to be at risk for the development of mental health problems. A Swedish large register study extending up to adulthood reported a three- to fourfold risk for mental health disorder leading to hospitalization (Hjern, Lindblad, & Vinnerljung, 2002), a fourfold risk of suicide (von Borczyskowski, Hjern, Lindblad, & Vinnerljung, 2006), and a fivefold risk for substance abuse among adopted children (Hjern, Lindblad, & Vinnerljung, 2002) when compared to nonadopted peers. The problem in the adoption studies, however, is that very rarely there has been any information on the conditions prior to adoption, leaving then considerable variance in the experience of ELS in different countries and during different historical circumstances. It is also unclear whether the nonadopted peers in the new homeland are the right comparison group for the adopted children, the results may be opposite if we compared them to their peers in their initial homeland, or to peers that remained in the institution. This is exactly what was done in the only randomized experiment among adopted children that was conducted in Romania. In that study, institutionalized children were randomly allocated either to foster care or to institutional care as usual. The results show family placement was an effective intervention which protected children from cognitive deficits (Nelson et al., 2007) and mental health problems (Zeanah et al., 2009) in their early development.

NATURAL EXPERIMENTS IN THE STUDY OF ELS

Another prominent way to study the effects of ELS on later mental health is to profit from the opportunities provided by experiments of nature. These happen, when unfortunate circumstances cause ELS randomly to some children, whereas their fellow peers remain intact. We are aware of three such natural experiments, which have examined the effects of ELS on later mental health with relatively long follow-up periods. The first is a study that examined the mental health of individuals placed immediately after birth into a Christmas Seal Home for an average period of seven months to avoid any contact with a mother with tuberculosis or any other family member. This prevention program against morbidity and mortality for tuberculosis in children was done with maternal consent and became an accepted public health policy, applying all social groups in Finland during the 1930s. In this register study, heightened risks for depression (Veijola et al., 2004), substance abuse (Veijola et al., 2008), and criminal behavior (Mäki et al., 2003a) have been reported among the formerly institutionalized newborns. Noteworthy is that the risk for schizophrenia or the risk for psychoses was not increased (Mäki et al., 2003b).

The second line of natural experiments has followed the life of Holocaust survivors, although very rare, these studies have focused on the survivors that were children during the war. One such study showed that child survivors had higher PTSD symptom scores, higher depression, anxiety, somatization, and anger-hostility scores and lower quality of life (Amir & Lev-Wiesel, 2001, 2003). Another study reported higher prevalence rates of anxiety disorders, sleep disturbances, and emotional distress among a sample consisting mainly of child and adolescent survivors, the findings being independent of age during the Holocaust (Sharon, Levav, Brodsky, Shemesh, & Kohn, 2009).

The third line of experimental research on ELS, which we have followed, is the examination the life course of children, who were evacuated from Finland during World War II to live with foster families in safer environments. Prior to development of Bowlby's attachment theory, in the late 1930s and early 1940s, there was not much theoretical understanding of the role of early attachment for later development. Yet, already in 1939, Bowlby, Miller, and Winnicott (1939) wrote a warning letter to the British Medical Journal noting the psychological cost that maternal separations could create:

> From among much research done on this subject a recent investigation carried out by one of us at the London Child Guidance Clinic may be quoted. It showed that one important external factor in the causation of persistent delinquency is a small child's prolonged separation from his mother. Over half of a statistically valid series of cases investigated had suffered periods of separation from their others and familiar environment lasting six months or more during their first five years of life. Study of individual case histories confirmed the statistical inference that the separation was the outstanding etiological factor in these cases. Apart from such a gross abnormality as chronic delinquency, mild behavior disorders, anxiety, and a tendency to vague physical illness can often be traced to such disturbances of the little child's environment, and most mothers of small children recognize this by being unwilling to leave their little children for more than very short

periods. . . . But the point that we wish to make is that such an experience in the case of a little child can mean far more than the actual experience of sadness. It can in fact amount to an emotional " black-out," and can easily lead to a severe disturbance of the development of the personality which may persist throughout life. (Orphans and children without homes start off as tragedies, and we are not dealing with the problems of their evacuation in this letter.) If these opinions are correct it follows that evacuation of small children without their mothers can lead to very serious and wide-spread psychological disorder. . . . A great deal more can be said about this problem on the basis of known facts. By this letter we only wish to draw the attention of those who are in authority to the existence of the problem. (pp. 1202–1203)

Despite this effort to draw the attention of policy makers, large-scale evacuations were organized in the United Kingdom and Finland. This created then an exceptional opportunity for contemporary psychology to study long-term lifespan outcomes related to parent–child separation in a natural setting, involving children from varying socioeconomic backgrounds. With regard to previous research, we are aware of only four studies in the United Kingdom, all based on the evacuation of children living in London during World War II, that have examined the long-term mental health outcomes of separation from both parents. The results are contradictory; one study found that former evacuees were more likely to have insecure attachment styles and lower levels of current psychological well-being than controls at the age of 67 years (Foster, Davies, & Steele, 2003). Two other studies, however, found no differences in adult mental health, depression and anxiety states between the former evacuees and the controls (Birtchnell & Kennard, 1984; Tennant, Hurry, & Bebbington, 1982). A more recent study (Rusby & Tasker, 2009), on the contrary, found that the former evacuees were in greater risk for depression and clinical anxiety. However, based on these studies, the evidence on the long-term consequences of parental separation is rather tenuous because of the small sample sizes, participant recruitment through advertisement and word of mouth, ambiguity related to the age when the outcomes were measured, paternal death in the control group, and data being partly restricted to women (Birtchnell & Kennard, 1984; Foster et al., 2003; Rusby & Tasker, 2009; Tennant et al., 1982).

Consequently, more research is needed to shed light on the life span consequences of ELS in humans. In the present chapter, we review our findings regarding the Finnish experience of evacuations in World War II. After providing background information on the study we review our empirical studies on war evacuees, followed by a general discussion.

CHILD EVACUATIONS IN THE HELSINKI BIRTH COHORT STUDY

During World War II, Finland fought two wars with the Soviet Union: the Winter War from November 1939 until March 1940 and the Continuation War from June 1941 until September 1944. To protect Finnish children from the effects of these wars, children from various socioeconomic backgrounds were evacuated abroad, primarily to Sweden and Denmark, unaccompanied by their parents. War strains were diverse and changed during the 1939–1940 war, and again in 1944, when the country experienced frequent air raids. There was also the threat of occupation by the enemy, which, however, never materialized. In 1942 food shortages were common, but there was also widespread expectation that the war would end soon. Since the evacuations were voluntary, the likelihood of a Finnish child being evacuated was influenced by an unpredictable interplay between political and familial factors (Kavén, 1985; Pesonen et al., 2007b). It is also of note that siblings were usually placed in different foster families to promote faster learning of the new language.

The evacuations had strong political support. Public criticism of the evacuations was discouraged by the government, and the media was used effectively to advocate the evacuations. Ultimately, the evacuations were seen as a positive opportunity in many families, particularly in 1942, when food shortages were severe and the war was expected to end soon (Kavén, 1985; Lomu, 1974). However, the war continued, and altogether approximately 70,000 children were sent into foster care unaccompanied by their parents for an average of almost two years (Kavén, 1985; Lomu, 1974; Pesonen et al., 2007a, 2007b). The Finnish National Archives preserve full documentation of the 48,628 children evacuated abroad by the Finnish government, the remaining 20,000 evacuations being organized by parents themselves.

The Helsinki Birth Cohort Study (HBCS) comprises 13,345 women ($n = 6,370$) and men ($n = 6,975$) who were born as singletons in one of the two main maternity hospitals in Helsinki, Finland, between 1934–1944, and who were living in Finland in 1971 when a unique personal identification number was allocated to each member of the Finnish population (Barker, Osmond, Forsén, Kajantie, & Eriksson, 2005). From the documents retrieved from the Finnish National Archives' register, we identified 1,781 (13.4% of the HBCS; $n = 822$, 46.2% women) participants who were separated temporarily from their parents as children. The register gives full documentation of all the children evacuated without their biological parents to temporary foster care abroad, mainly in Sweden and

Denmark, through the Ministry of Social Affairs and Health between 1939 and 1946. The age at the time of separation (M = 4.7 years, SD = 2.4 years) and the duration of the separation (M = 1.7 years, SD = 1.0 years) were also identified from the register. In the study of ELS on subsequent life, we have thus profited from this register-based information on ELS, which allowed a very accurate examination of the effects of duration and timing of ELS on later well-being.

Given that many of the evacuations were not registered, our first studies on evacuations (Pesonen et al., 2007a, 2008) were conducted in a subsample of the HBCS, of whom we had questionnaire-based information on parental separations in addition to the information derived from the register. From the questionnaire, we were able to identify additional individuals separated from both their parents during the war who were not registered in the Finnish National Archives. In later studies, however, we rely exclusively on the register data. However, we excluded from the analyses the few cases (n = 189) reported to be separated in the questionnaire but not registered in the Finnish National Archives.

FINDINGS ON DEPRESSIVE SYMPTOMS

One of our first studies was conducted in a subsample of the HBCS. This subsample was randomly selected from the initial cohort. They underwent detailed clinical examination on cardiometabolic and hormonal characteristics and filled in a survey including depressive symptoms in 2001–2003 and 2004. Thus, our first study on the separated children was based on 1,658 participants of the HBCS, who had filled in the Beck Depression Inventory twice, an average two years apart (Pesonen et al., 2007a). We found that those who had been separated as children unaccompanied by either parent to temporary foster care reported, at the average age of approximately 60 years, 20% more severe depressive symptoms than did those who did not experience any parental separation in times of war. Furthermore, they were almost twice as likely to remain at least mild in severity in depressive symptoms over two consecutive measurement occasions in late adulthood. Moreover, separation that lasted more than three years had the largest effect, being associated with over 33% more severe depressive symptoms, with an odds ratio of 4.4 for belonging to the group who reported depressive symptoms remaining at least mild in severity over time. Finally, those who had been separated either in infancy or at school age reported over 23% and 30% more severe depressive symptoms in late adulthood, whereas those separated in toddlerhood (aged from two to four years) or in early childhood (aged from four to six years) seemed to be the least affected.

With regard to the contradictory data derived from the British experience of evacuations, we argued that our results may be more reliable. Unlike the British studies, our study was based on an epidemiologic cohort and data on separations were mainly based on register information. In addition, we were able to test our hypotheses in larger samples, and with a well-validated measure of depression. However, our study had also limitations that are in common with our other studies on this subject. First, although children were evacuated from all socioeconomic backgrounds, it was more likely that children in the lowest category of socioeconomic status (SES) became separated. Although we controlled for childhood and adulthood SES in all our analyses, its role should not be overlooked. For instance, there is always the possibility that the decision to evacuate the child was dependent on family adversity other than that related to measurable SES, such adversity acting as a potential confounder. Secondly, we do not have information on the quality of foster care, which, of course, could have modified the stress experience of the children (Rusby & Tasker, 2009).

FINDINGS ON PSYCHIATRIC MORBIDITY AND MORTALITY

We have preliminary data on the mental health of the former evacuees from the entire birth cohort with available data, involving 12,747 participants (96% of the initial cohort), of whom 1,719 had been separated according to the register information (Räikkönen et al., 2010). This study examined the cumulative incidence of psychiatric disorders from early to late adulthood severe enough to require hospital treatment or cause death in the separated and the nonseparated. Diagnoses on psychiatric disorders from early to late adulthood and severe enough to require hospital treatment were identified from the Finnish Hospital Discharge Register (HDR), and severe enough to cause death from the Finnish Causes of Death Register (CDR).

The first findings indicate that compared to the nonseparated, the separated showed a higher cumulative incidence of any psychiatric disorders, and of substance use and personality disorder. We also found that individuals with an upper childhood socioeconomic background were particularly sensitive to the temporary separations and showed the highest cumulative incidence psychiatric disorders. The associations were not specific to age at or length of the temporal separations, and were not confounded by factors that were associated with a higher likelihood of being temporarily separated from the parents and/or that may pose a risk for later psychiatric disorders.

The findings linking temporary separation from the parents specifically with substance use and personality disorders, but not with psychoses are, thus, in agreement with the previous findings (Johnson, Cohen, Brown, Smailes, & Bernstein, 1999; Mäki et al., 2003a; Veijola et al., 2008; Widom, Czaja, & Paris, 2009; Widom, DuMont, & Czaja, 2007; Widom, Ireland, & Glynn, 1995), but our null findings with mood and anxiety disorders were discordant with past reports (Danese et al., 2009; Mäkikyrö et al., 1998; Veijola et al., 2008; Widom et al., 2007). Yet, we previously reported that the temporary separations from the parents were associated with depressive symptoms in a subsample of the current study (Pesonen et al., 2007a).

FINDINGS ON STRESS REACTIVITY

Animal models have demonstrated that consequences of ELS may lead to physiological changes in the central nervous system that may be permanent. Among the plausible physiological mechanisms behind the associations is of ELS and later psychiatric morbidity is stress-related hypothalamic-pituitary-adrenal (HPA) axis functioning that shows associations with a number of psychiatric disorders (Claes, 2004). Animals who have experienced ELS show increased corticotrophin-releasing hormone expression and decreased numbers of glucocorticoid receptors in the hippocampus, hypothalamus, and frontal cortex (Ladd, Owens, & Nemeroff, 1996) and methylation of hippocampal glucocorticoid receptor genes (Weaver et al., 2001), all reflecting altered neural plasticity at multiple levels of the central nervous system. At a behavioral level, lower levels of glucocorticoid receptors have been associated with poorer stress regulation capacity and more prolonged stress reactions (Weaver et al., 2004). Consequently, early separated animals exhibit greater startle responses, greater freezing and anxiety responses, and two- to threefold greater hormonal responses to stress as adults (Cirulli, Berry, & Alleva, 2003).

We had the opportunity to study the hormonal stress reactivity of a subsample of the HBCS ($n = 282$), using the Trier Social Stress Test (TSST) (Pesonen et al., 2010). The TSST is a psychosocial stress test in which the subject is asked to give a speech and do a series of subtractions in front of the committee. This committee minimized all verbal and nonverbal communication with the subject in order to add stressfulness to the performance. This is a well-validated procedure that is known to elicit a powerful hormonal stress response (Kudielka, Buske-Kirschbaum, Hellhammer, & Kirschbaum, 2004; Kudielka, Schommer,

Hellhammer, & Kirschbaum, 2004), measured via cortisol in saliva and in plasma, and from plasma ACTH.

We found that ELS was associated with altered responsiveness of the HPA axis more than 60 years after childhood separation (Pesonen et al., 2010). In comparison to nonseparated individuals, individuals separated from both parents at a mean of three years of age displayed 20%–25% higher salivary cortisol and plasma ACTH levels across the time points during the TSST, and higher salivary cortisol reactivity in response to the TSST, more than 60 years later.

Importantly, altered stress reactivity can be due to current depressive symptoms, and not to initial trauma. Therefore, we controlled for the current depressive symptoms in our analyses, and found that the association between a childhood traumatic event and HPA axis function is not explained by the presence of symptoms of depression (Pesonen et al., 2010). This suggests that the interrelations between ELS, stress physiology, and mental health are not merely due to symptoms of depression. Rather, our findings may suggest that ELS may have "programmed" the function of the HPA axis: as the brain continues to develop after birth, brain development during childhood may be especially vulnerable a period for the effects of glucocorticoids. Perhaps ELS is one factor underlying the consistently documented association between altered HPA axis functioning and depression. Our observations accorded with previous studies showing that the association between ELS and HPA axis responsiveness are stronger among men than women (Tyrka, Wyche, Kelly, Price, & Carpenter, 2009). In addition, we observed an inverse U-shaped relationship between age at separation and both salivary or plasma cortisol and plasma ACTH reactivity. The highest concentrations were observed in the middle of the age range among the children separated from both parents, that is, among those separated as toddlers and in early childhood. Comparison of this observation to earlier observations is difficult, since the specific age period of ELS due to abusive experiences can rarely be identified retrospectively. Studies of parental loss or divorce, on the other hand, have not been able to specify age periods with such accuracy (Bloch, Peleg, Koren, Aner, & Klein, 2007; Luecken & Appelhans, 2006; Tyrka et al., 2009). It might have been that the children in the middle of the age range might have perceived the social and cultural upheavals of separation (foreign language and customs, new peers) as more difficult to cope with owing to their undeveloped self-regulative capacities, and this uncontrollability is associated with higher HPA axis responses later on. Significantly, the duration of separation did not have an independent effect on hormonal reactivity.

FINDINGS ON COGNITIVE ABILITY

Importantly, the neural circuitry of stress involves several brain structures, including the hippocampus, amygdala, and prefrontal cortex, all of which are vital to cognitive function. Indeed, animal research has suggested that ELS may also accelerate late-onset progressive impairment of the hippocampus and cognitive function (Brunson et al., 2005; Rice, Sandman, Lenjavi, & Baram, 2008). The human evidence, however, is scarce. It shows that institutionalized children, in comparison to their siblings or peers who were adopted from these institutions, obtained lower scores on tests of intellectual ability at an average age of 54 months (Nelson et al., 2007). When compared to peers in their new homeland, intercountry adoptees scored lower on tests of intellectual ability in young adulthood (Nelson et al., 2007; Odenstad et al., 2008; van Ijzendoorn, Juffer, & Poelhuis, 2005). Further, a recent study demonstrated that elderly Holocaust survivors had a greater age-related decline in explicit memory compared to their nonexposed peers (Yehuda et al., 2006). These studies can, however, rarely distinguish other factors accompanied by early stress, such as impaired nutrition.

Our preliminary results provide further prospective evidence on the long-term intellectual outcomes of ELS among 2,725 men of HBCS (Pesonen et al., submitted manuscript). Data on verbal, arithmetic, and visuospatial intellectual abilities of the young adults of the HBCS was retrieved from the archives of the Finnish Defence Forces: since the 1950s, every Finnish man has undergone this test in conjunction with his compulsory military service. This obligatory test is given to all new recruits during the first two weeks of their military service and is used when the conscripts are selected for leadership training. The test battery is designed to measure general ability and logical thinking, is composed of verbal, visuospatial, and arithmetic reasoning subtests. Each subtest is timed and consists of 40 multiple-choice questions that are ordered by difficulty. Correct answers are summed to yield a test score.

We found that the separated had −0.28 SD to −0.13 units lower verbal, visuospatial, and arithmetic ability scores, as compared to nonseparated individuals (Pesonen et al., submitted manuscript). Consistent to previous retrospective and scant prospective evidence, we found the strongest relationship between ELS and lower scores on verbal reasoning (Bremner, 2006; Saigh, Yasik, Oberfield, Halamandaris, & Bremner, 2006; Yasik, Saigh, Oberfield, & Halamandaris, 2007). The associations were not confounded by childhood social class, birth order, birth weight or by age or height at time of intellectual assessment, factors that previous research has found as predictors of intellectual development.

In addition we observed a threshold effect between duration of stress exposure and impairment of intellectual ability, such that a separation lasting for one year or less was not associated with worse intellectual performance. Second, we were able to specify an age period when the child is probably most vulnerable to ELS. The most widely affected children were aged from two to four years, and from four to seven years when first separated, whereas separation in infancy or at school age had fewer effects on the test scores, except for the verbal ability score. Our finding corresponds to our previous observation that the highest HPA axis reactivity to stress in adults occurs within this same group of separation age (Pesonen et al., 2010).

These findings showing that infancy may be a period of lesser vulnerability parallels findings showing that adoption during infancy may buffer the potentially adverse developmental consequences of institutionalization (Gunnar & van Dulmen, 2007; Nelson et al., 2007). However, the analogy may be misleading. Whereas earlier adoption is likely to reduce the potential time of social deprivation, we do not know whether the separated children were actually deprived in their foster families.

FINDINGS ON LIFE HISTORY

Targeting solely on mental health outcomes, stress reactivity, or cognitive ability, may not effectively describe the long-term consequences of ELS. Therefore, we also examined whether the separations were associated with reproductive and marital traits among a subsample of 1,704 former evacuees (Pesonen et al., 2008). According to the life history theory and its variations (Belsky, 2008; Charnov, 1993), a risky and uncertain environment during childhood may lead to reproducing early in life in order to maximize the probability of leaving descents. Among humans, this theory is supported by fairly rich retrospective evidence associating general childhood family adversities, or the father's absence, with an earlier onset of menarche (Ellis, 2005). Among the few existing prospective studies, a recent large-scale one showed that children who were adopted in Denmark had a 10–20 times greater risk for developing a precocious puberty compared to inhabitants of Danish origin (Teilmann, Pedersen, Skakkebaek, & Jensen, 2006). While most of the existing evidence points to earlier rather than later pubertal development, there are data from the former Yugoslavia (Prebeg & Bralic, 2000), suggesting delayed pubertal development in times of the war, at least in girls exposed to stressful conditions during or shortly before their menarcheal age. Our aim was to test whether a separation in childhood was associated with reproductive traits later in life, measured by age at onset of menarche. We also explored the associations between a separation and age at first childbirth, number of children by late adulthood and their interbirth intervals, all issues which have not been prospectively tested against a childhood psychosocial trauma in an epidemiological cohort (Pesonen et al., 2008).

In accordance with earlier studies, we found that the separated women had an earlier onset of menarche than nonseparated women, independent of the year of birth, mothers' age at menarche, childhood SES, and Body Mass Index at age seven (Pesonen et al., 2008). Compared to the nonseparated girls, the separated girls were 2.1 times more likely to have their menarche before or at the age of 12 than after the age of 13. An adjustment for general parental quality during, measured by a retrospective report childhood did not affect the results, further emphasizing the role of separation in explaining the results. We also found that the separated women had given birth to more children than the nonseparated women. Compared to the nonseparated women, the separated women were 2.3 times more likely to have four or more children, and 1.9 times more likely to have three children than to have a single child. The findings concerned also men: the separated men had their first child at a younger age than the nonseparated men, and the interbirth intervals were shorter. Based on these observations, we hypothesized that a traumatic experience may lead to a need to start a family at an earlier age in order to overcome the instability derived from the trauma. Even though the effects were relatively weak, they were theoretically based and delineated a consistent tendency to maximize early reproduction in uncertain times, such as following childhood psychosocial trauma. In agreement with recent theorizing (Belsky, 2008), instead of emphasizing nonoptimal, development disruptions, the results clearly challenge to put more emphasis on considering the adaptive life solutions following the trauma-related coping processes.

Finally, we also tested whether the ELS had consequences on marital history of the evacuees. Contrary to general expectations, we found that separation associated with smaller likelihood to divorce later in life, both in men and women. We do not know, however, whether this finding reflected heightened marital satisfaction, or whether it reflected increased attachment anxiety, an excessive concern about abandonment, which may function as a maintaining force for proximity even in unhappy marriages (Davila & Bradbury, 2001).

GENERAL COMMENTS

As recently summarized (Gunnar & Fisher, 2006), the major challenges in human studies on ELS are to get as close as possible to experimental conditions and to obtain more information on the timing of trauma. Our study in the HBSC unique natural experimental setting, of which approximately 13% were exposed to a specific form of ELS, parental separation, has allowed us to overcome some of the challenges relating to human studies on ELS. These kinds of exceptional conditions are particularly significant to natural experimental designs because potential confounders are assumed to be randomly distributed across the groups under investigation. Thus, we have argued that the likelihood of a Finnish child being evacuated was at some extent random, influenced by an unpredictable interplay between political and intrafamilial factors, such as the parents generally choosing to send only one or some children away. In 1942, when the first massive wave of evacuations took place, the war was also expected to end quickly. Even child mental health professionals in Finland advocated the evacuations, creating the sense that this was an opportunity for children, as Finnish child psychiatrist T. Brander pertinently remarked in 1943 (Brander, 1943):

> Not a single case has come to my attention in which a child suffered psychological injury from this voluntary evacuation. Quite the contrary: such a stay proved to be an instructive and refreshing experience, from which the children returned with heightened vitality. This was due to the excellent care and attention bestowed on our children by our western neighbors. (p. 314)

However, several methodological considerations should be taken account when interpreting the findings. In the studies among subsamples of the HBCS, investigating the associations between depressive symptoms and stress reactivity, we found the differences in the socioeconomic background of the separated and nonseparated were not statistically significant. However, in studies involving more subjects, we observed a statistically significant difference in childhood SES: the separated originated more frequently from lower socioeconomic background. Although we have adjusted for childhood SES in all our studies, the role of childhood SES on later outcomes may have been more complex, thus acting as a potential confounder in our studies. On the other hand, when we examined the role of ELS in later psychiatric morbidity and mortality, it was especially those participants who originated from upper socioeconomic position that were in increased risk for later psychiatric disorders, whereas the temporary separations did not add to the risk otherwise associated with a lower childhood socioeconomic background. In this sense, preponderance of separation in the lowest category of childhood SES may have even masked the effects of ELS in our studies. In addition, our findings suggested that an upper childhood socioeconomic background may not buffer from severe ELS, such as that arising from temporary separations from parents.

Another challenge in the longitudinal studies is the sampling bias. Those who responded to the depression questionnaire may have been healthier than those who did not, and those who attended the stressful stress test may have been more adventurous and less depressed than those who refused. This kind of sampling bias concerned only these two studies based on voluntary participation. A second source of sampling bias is related to the migration processes and childhood mortality, thus concerning all our studies. Approximately 11% of the separated were adopted in Sweden as child. However, a previous study (Räsänen, 1992) found no significant differences in mental health status between the adopted and returned former child evacuees. In addition to adoptions, the migration processes between Sweden and Finland have been relatively complex, some adopted children moving back to Finland as they grew up, and some former evacuees moving back to Sweden as young adults. Noteworthy, the emigration in adulthood was more likely for former child evacuees than for the nonseparated in the HBCS (Räikkönen et al., submitted manuscript). The mortality of evacuated children was 0.6% over the whole evacuation period (mean: 2.1 years), slightly lower than the annual mortality among Finnish children aged one to nine years, which ranged from 0.4% to 0.5% during 1941–1945 (Pesonen et al., 2007a). We also acknowledge that the parents may have generally chosen the weakest children, causing potential bias. However, the original governmental policy aimed at excluding unhealthy children. Later in the war, sick children (11% of registered evacuations, 3.5% mortality) were also considered eligible for evacuation (Pesonen et al., 2007a).

Finally, we are aware that evacuated children may have experienced other adversities during their foreign stay, making it difficult to isolate the effect of separation from other influences. However, we definitely know that the children lost their secure base with the unpredictable evacuation and, thus, also lost the parental assistance needed in regulating emotions, especially under serious stress. As a subjective case report describes (Serenius, 1995), the separation trauma evoked both dissociative memory function and uncontrollable anxiety, which characterized individual emotion regulation even 50 years after evacuation.

In conclusion, our study presents evidence of long-term mental health disadvantage and cognitive impairment following experience of ELS.

Although the historical circumstances in this study were particular, the developmental significance of ELS is not bound to this study. According to data reported by the United Nations Refugee Agency (UNHCR) in 2008, there were 42 million displaced individuals worldwide, including 15.2 refugees, of which 44% are children (http://www.unhcr.org/4a375c426. html). Even without displacement, an experience of ELS for various reasons, parental loss or family disruption, child abuse and neglect, traumatizing events, illness, poverty, institutionalization, or war concerns children everywhere in the contemporary world.

REFERENCES

Alastalo, H., Räikkönen, K., Pesonen, A. K., Osmond, C., Barker, D. J., Kajantie, E., et al. (2009). Cardiovascular health of Finnish war evacuees 60 years later. *Annals of Medicine, 41*, 66–72.

Amir, M., & Lev-Wiesel, R. (2001). Does everyone have a name? Psychological distress and quality of life among child Holocaust survivors with lost identity. *Journal of Traumatic Stress, 14*, 859–869.

Amir, M., & Lev-Wiesel, R. (2003). Time does not heal all wounds: Quality of life and psychological distress of people who survived the Holocaust as children 55 years later. *Journal of Traumatic Stress, 16*, 295–299.

Barker, D. J., Osmond, C., Forsén, T. J., Kajantie, E., & Eriksson, J. G. (2005). Trajectories of growth among children who have coronary events as adults. *New England Journal of Medicine, 353*, 1802–1809.

Belsky, J. (2008). War, trauma and children's development: Observations from a modern evolutionary perspective. *International Journal of Behavioral Development, 32*, 260–271.

Birtchnell, J., & Kennard, J. (1984). How do the experiences of the early separated and the early bereaved differ and to what extent do such differences affect outcome? *Social Psychiatry, 19*, 163–171.

Bloch, M., Peleg, I., Koren, D., Aner, H., & Klein, E. (2007). Long-term effects of early parental loss due to divorce on the HPA axis. *Hormones and Behavior, 51*, 516–523.

Bowlby, J., Miller, E., & Winnicott, D. W. (1939). Evacuation of small children. *British Medical Journal, 2*(4119), 1202–1203.

Brander, T. (1943). Psychiatric observations among Finnish children during Russo-Finnish war of 1939–1940. *Nervous Child, 2*, 313–319.

Bremner, J. D. (2006). Traumatic stress: Effects on the brain. *Dialogues in Clinical Neuroscience, 8*, 445–461.

Brunson, K. L., Kramar, E., Lin, B., Chen, Y., Colgin, L. L., Yanagihara, T. K., et al. (2005). Mechanisms of late-onset cognitive decline after early-life stress. *Journal of Neuroscience, 25*, 9328–9338.

Charnov, E. L. (1993). *Life history invariants*. Oxford: Oxford University Press.

Cirulli, F., Berry, A., & Alleva, E. (2003). Early disruption of the mother–infant relationship: Effects on brain plasticity and implications for psychopathology. *Neuroscience and Biobehavioral Reviews, 27*, 73–82.

Claes, S. J. (2004). Corticotropin-releasing hormone (CRH) in psychiatry: From stress to psychopathology. *Annals of Medicine, 36*, 50–61.

Danese, A., Moffitt, T. E., Harrington, H., Milne, B. J., Polanczyk, G., Pariante, C. M., et al. (2009). Adverse childhood experiences and adult risk factors for age-related disease: Depression, inflammation, and clustering of metabolic risk markers. *Archives of Pediatric and Adolescent Medicine, 163*, 1135–1143.

Danese, A., Moffitt, T. E., Pariante, C. M., Ambler, A., Poulton, R., & Caspi, A. (2008). Elevated inflammation levels in depressed adults with a history of childhood maltreatment. *Archives of General Psychiatry, 65*, 409–415.

Davila, J., & Bradbury, T. N. (2001). Attachment insecurity and the distinction between unhappy spouses who do and do not divorce. *Journal of Family Psychology, 15*, 371–393.

Ellis, B. J. (2005). Determinants of pubertal timing: An evolutionary developmental approach. In B.J.B.D.F. Ellis (Ed.), *Origins of the social mind: Evolutionary psychology and child development* (pp. 164–188). New York: Guilford Press.

Foster, D., Davies, S., & Steele, H. (2003). The evacuation of British children during World War II: A preliminary investigation into the long-term psychological effects. *Aging and Mental Health, 7*, 398–408.

Gunnar, M., & Fisher, P. A. (2006). Bringing basic research on early experience and stress neurobiology to bear on preventive interventions for neglected and maltreated children. *Development and Psychopathology, 18*, 651–677.

Gunnar, M., & Quevedo, K. (2007). The neurobiology of stress and development. *Annual Review of Psychology, 58*, 145–173.

Gunnar, M., & van Dulmen, M. H. (2007). Behavior problems in postinstitutionalized internationally adopted children. *Development and Psychopathology, 19*, 129–148.

Hjern, A., Lindblad, F., & Vinnerljung, B. (2002). Suicide, psychiatric illness, and social maladjustment in intercountry adoptees in Sweden: A cohort study. *The Lancet, 360*, 443–448.

Holmes, A., le Guisquet, A. M., Vogel, E., Millstein, R. A., Leman, S., & Belzung, C. (2005). Early life genetic, epigenetic and environmental factors shaping emotionality in rodents. *Neuroscience and Biobehavioral Reviews, 29*, 1335–1346.

Johnson, J. G., Cohen, P., Brown, J., Smailes, E. M., & Bernstein, D. P. (1999). Childhood maltreatment increases risk for personality disorders during early adulthood. *Archives of General Psychiatry, 56*, 600–606.

Kavén, P. (1985). *70 000 pientä kohtaloa*. Helsinki: Otava.

Kudielka, B. M., Buske-Kirschbaum, A., Hellhammer, D. H., & Kirschbaum, C. (2004). HPA axis responses to laboratory psychosocial stress in healthy elderly adults, younger adults, and children: Impact of age and gender. *Psychoneuroendocrinology, 29*, 83–98.

Kudielka, B. M., Schommer, N. C., Hellhammer, D. H., & Kirschbaum, C. (2004). Acute HPA axis responses, heart rate, and mood changes to psychosocial stress (TSST) in humans at different times of day. *Psychoneuroendocrinology, 29*, 983–992.

Ladd, C. O., Owens, M. J., & Nemeroff, C. B. (1996). Persistent changes in corticotropin-releasing factor neuronal systems induced by maternal deprivation. *Endocrinology, 137*, 1212–1218.

Lomu, J. (1974). *Lastensiirtokomitea ja sen arkisto 1941–1949* [The committee of child evacuations 1941–1949] (Archival Code 441:5). Helsinki: Finnish National Archives.

Luecken, L. J., & Appelhans, B. M. (2006). Early parental loss and salivary cortisol in young adulthood: The moderating role of family environment. *Development and Psychopathology, 18*, 295–308.

Mäki, P., Veijola, J., Joukamaa, M., Läärä, E., Hakko, H., Jones, P. B., et al. (2003a). Maternal separation at birth and schizophrenia—a long-term follow-up of the Finnish Christmas Seal Home Children. *Schizophrenia Research, 60*, 13–19.

Mäki, P., Veijola, J., Räsänen, P., Joukamaa, M., Valonen, P., Jokelainen, J., et al. (2003b). Criminality in the offspring of antenatally depressed mothers: A 33-year follow-up of the Northern Finland 1966 Birth Cohort. *Journal of Affective Disorders, 74*, 273–278.

Mäkikyrö, T., Sauvola, A., Moring, J., Veijola, J., Nieminen, P., Järvelin, M. R., et al. (1998). Hospital-treated psychiatric disorders in adults with a single-parent and two-parent family background: A 28-year follow-up of the 1966 Northern Finland Birth Cohort. *Family Processes, 37*, 335–344.

Nelson, C. A., III, Zeanah, C. H., Fox, N. A., Marshall, P. J., Smyke, A. T., & Guthrie, D. (2007). Cognitive recovery in socially deprived young children: The Bucharest Early Intervention Project. *Science, 318*, 1937–1940.

Odenstad, A., Hjern, A., Lindblad, F., Rasmussen, F., Vinnerljung, B., & Dalen, M. (2008). Does age at adoption and geographic origin matter? A national cohort study of cognitive test performance in adult inter-country adoptees. *Psychological Medicine, 38*, 1803–1814.

Pesonen, A. K., Räikkönen, K., Feldt, K., Heinonen, K., Osmond, C., Phillips, D.I.W., et al. (2010). Childhood traumatic separation experience predicts hormonal response at age 60 to 70: A natural experiment in World War II. *Psychoneuroendocrinology, 35*, 758–767.

Pesonen, A. K., Räikkönen, K., Heinonen, K., Kajantie, E., Forsén, T., & Eriksson, J. G. (2007a). Depressive symptoms in adults separated from their parents as children: A natural experiment during World War II. *American Journal of Epidemiology, 166*, 1126–1133.

Pesonen, A. K., Räikkönen, K., Heinonen, K., Kajantie, E., Forsén, T., & Eriksson, J. G. (2007b). Pesonen et al. respond to "The life course epidemiology of depression." *American Journal of Epidemiology, 166,* 1138–1139.

Pesonen, A. K., Räikkönen, K., Heinonen, K., Kajantie, E., Forsén, T., & Eriksson, J. G. (2008). Reproductive traits following a parent–child separation trauma during childhood: A natural experiment during World War II. *American Journal of Human Biology, 20*, 345–351.

Prebeg, Z., & Bralic, I. (2000). Changes in menarcheal age in girls exposed to war conditions. *American Journal of Human Biology, 12*, 503–508.

Pryce, C. R., Ruedi-Bettschen, D., Dettling, A. C., Weston, A., Russig, H., Ferger, B., et al. (2005). Long-term effects of early-life environmental manipulations in rodents and primates: Potential animal models in depression research. *Neuroscience and Biobehavioral Reviews, 29*, 649–674.

Räikkönen, K., Lahti , M., Heinonen, K., Pesonen, A. K., Wahlbeck, K., Kajantie, E., et al. (2010). Risk of severe mental disorders in adults separated temporarily from their parents in childhood: The Helsinki birth cohort study. *Journal of Psychiatric Research*.

Räsänen, E. (1992). Excessive life changes during childhood and their effects on mental and physical health in adulthood. *Acta Paedopsychiatr, 55*, 19–24.

Rice, C. J., Sandman, C. A., Lenjavi, M. R., & Baram, T. Z. (2008). A novel mouse model for acute and long-lasting consequences of early life stress. *Endocrinology, 149*, 4892–4900.

Rusby, J. S., & Tasker, F. (2009). Long-term effects of the British evacuation of children during World War 2 on their adult mental health. *Aging Ment Health, 13*, 391–404.

Saigh, P. A., Yasik, A. E., Oberfield, R. A., Halamandaris, P. V., & Bremner, J. D. (2006). The intellectual performance of traumatized children and adolescents with or without posttraumatic stress disorder. *Journal of Abnormal Psychology, 115*, 332–340.

Serenius, M. (1995). The silent cry: A Finnish child during World War II and 50 years later. *International Forum of Psychoanalysis, 4*, 35–47.

Sharon, A., Levav, I., Brodsky, J., Shemesh, A. A., & Kohn, R. (2009). Psychiatric disorders and other health dimensions among Holocaust survivors 6 decades later. *British Journal Psychiatry, 195*, 331–335.

Teilmann, G., Pedersen, C. B., Skakkebaek, N. E., & Jensen, T. K. (2006). Increased risk of precocious puberty in internationally adopted children in Denmark. *Pediatrics, 118*, e391–399.

Tennant, C., Hurry, J., & Bebbington, P. (1982). The relation of childhood separation experiences to adult depressive and anxiety states. *British Journal of Psychiatry, 141*, 475–482.

Tyrka, A. R., Wyche, M. C., Kelly, M. M., Price, L. H., & Carpenter, L. L. (2009). Childhood maltreatment and adult personality disorder symptoms: Influence of maltreatment type. *Psychiatry Research, 165*, 281–287.

van Ijzendoorn, M. H., Juffer, F., & Poelhuis, C. W. (2005). Adoption and cognitive development: A meta-analytic comparison of adopted and nonadopted children's IQ and school performance. *Psychological Bulletin, 131*, 301–316.

Veijola, J., Läärä, E., Joukamaa, M., Isohanni, M., Hakko, H., Haapea, M., et al. (2008). Temporary parental separation at birth and substance use disorder in adulthood: A long-term follow-up of the Finnish Christmas Seal Home Children. *Social Psychiatry and Psychiatric Epidemiology, 43*, 11–17.

Veijola, J., Mäki, P., Joukamaa, M., Läärä, E., Hakko, H., & Isohanni, M. (2004). Parental separation at birth and depression in adulthood: A long-term follow-up of the Finnish Christmas Seal Home Children. *Psychological Medicine, 34*, 357–362.

von Borczyskowski, A., Hjern, A., Lindblad, F., & Vinnerljung, B. (2006). Suicidal behaviour in national and international adult adoptees: A Swedish cohort study. *Social Psychiatry and Psychiatric Epidemiology, 41*, 95–102.

Weaver, I. C., Cervoni, N., Champagne, F. A., D'Alessio, A. C., Sharma, S., Seckl, J. R., et al. (2004). Epigenetic programming by maternal behavior. *Nature Neuroscience, 7*, 847–854.

Weaver, I. C., La Plante, P., Weaver, S., Parent, A., Sharma, S., Diorio, J., et al. (2001). Early environmental regulation of hippocampal glucocorticoid receptor gene expression: Characterization of intracellular mediators and potential genomic target sites. *Molecular and Cellular Endocrinology, 185*, 205–218.

Widom, C. S., Czaja, S. J., & Paris, J. (2009). A prospective investigation of borderline personality disorder in abused and neglected children followed up into adulthood. *Journal of Personality Disorders, 23*, 433–446.

Widom, C. S., DuMont, K., & Czaja, S. J. (2007). A prospective investigation of major depressive disorder and comorbidity in abused and neglected children grown up. *Archives of General Psychiatry, 64*, 49–56.

Widom, C. S., Ireland, T., & Glynn, P. J. (1995). Alcohol abuse in abused and neglected children followed-up: Are they at increased risk? *Journal of Studies on Alcohol, 56*, 207–217.

Yasik, A. E., Saigh, P. A., Oberfield, R. A., & Halamandaris, P. V. (2007). Posttraumatic stress disorder: Memory and learning performance in children and adolescents. *Biological Psychiatry, 61*, 382–388.

Yehuda, R., Tischler, L., Golier, J. A., Grossman, R., Brand, S. R., Kaufman, S., et al. (2006). Longitudinal assessment of cognitive performance in Holocaust survivors with and without PTSD. *Biological Psychiatry, 60*, 714–721.

Zeanah, C. H., Egger, H. L., Smyke, A. T., Nelson, C. A., Fox, N. A., Marshall, P. J., et al. (2009). Institutional rearing and psychiatric disorders in Romanian preschool children. *American Journal of Psychiatry, 166*, 777–785.

Chapter 10

CHILDREN SEEKING ASYLUM: THE PSYCHOLOGICAL AND DEVELOPMENTAL IMPACT OF THE REFUGEE EXPERIENCE

Louise Newman

At the end of 2008 the United Nations High Commissioner for Refugees (UNHCR) estimated that there were 10 million refugees around the world and over 14 million internally displaced persons. Many more were deemed stateless (over 6 million), with a total of 34 million "of concern" to the agency. Around one-third of these persons were children aged 6–17 years, and around 10% were less than five years of age. Infants and children constitute a significant proportion of those impacted by war, conflict, displacement and loss and are among the most vulnerable.

The developed world maintains a clear approach aimed at regulating and limiting the influx of asylum seekers and there remains community concern about the impact of new arrivals on employment, standard of life and cultural values. The term *multiculturalism* has become highly charged for some nations and also highly politicized. Pressure increased during the 1990s with increasing numbers of displaced persons seeking asylum in response to war and mass violations of human rights (UNHCR, 2000). Many had experienced torture, sexual assault and other trauma and presented with a range of health and mental health issues. Children have been both witness to and direct victims of atrocity (Murthy & Lakshminarayana, 2006).

In spite of the overwhelming needs of asylum seeking people the majority of industrialized countries have no formal resettlement programs with the result that millions of people seek asylum directly with some entering countries in an "unauthorized" fashion (around 5 million from 1995 to

2001). Humanitarian protection programs are limited with many refugees spending protracted periods in refugee camps and being further exposed to deprivation and trauma. The main response of many rich nations has been to develop so-called policies of "deterrence," including increasing border protection measures and limiting rights to appeal (Silove, Steel, & Walters, 2000). In some countries, particularly Australia, asylum seekers have had limited access to health care, education and work rights. These restrictive measures directly impact the welfare, development, and health of infants and children and have been particularly controversial.

Perhaps the most controversial measure introduced in some countries has been the detention of asylum seekers, including women, infants and children. The United States, United Kingdom, Germany, Italy, and Australia have all detained significant numbers of children as routine practice despite concerns about the nature of detention environments and difficulties providing child support, activities, and education. The practice of detaining children, including unaccompanied minors as well as those with family groups, seems to be in conflict with the statements of the UNHCR that detention of children should only be used as a measure of last resort and for short periods of time. The housing of family groups in immigration detention facilities creates specific management difficulties and raises issues as to how best to protect the human rights of children in this situation. In the United States more than 5,000 children are held in immigration detention on an annual basis and in 2006 a 512-bed facility purpose built for the detention of families was opened in Texas. The British government has formally submitted a reservation to the UNHCR seeking to enable children subject to immigration control to be excluded from human rights provisions (Newman & Steel, 2008). Australia was the first developed nation to develop a policy of mandatory detention for all "unauthorized" arrivals and allowed this for an indefinite period time (Silove, Austin, & Steel, 2007). Detention of children has highlighted what may be seen as a fundamental tension between the priorities of immigration law and the rights of children to care and protection.

Although voluntary signatories to the United Nations Convention on the Rights of the Child, it is arguable that several countries stand in breach of this and related conventions in an ongoing way. In Australia, for example, the use of a remote facility for processing of asylum seekers on Christmas Island, in effect detains all child asylum seekers and does not allow for community detention placements of families with infants and children (Newman, 2009). In the midst of debates about the appropriate response to asylum seekers, infants and children have become caught in a system that is unable to provide adequate protection or support for those who have already experienced significant trauma. The following discussion will review the psychological and developmental impact of immigration detention on child asylum seekers, with reference to the Australian experience and research findings.

SEEKING ASYLUM, DETENTION, AND MENTAL HEALTH

Between 1999 and 2005 around 3,000 children were held in immigration detention facilities in Australia. The average length of stay in 2003 was around 20 months. Significant numbers of unaccompanied minors, mainly adolescent boys, were also detained. Detention facilities were in remote regions with little provision for the health and mental health needs of detainees, and in particular, limited facilities for children and inadequate play and educational services—in effect, a neglectful environment. In addition to environmental and emotional deprivation, children were also impacted by the experiences of their parents/caregivers, many of whom developed significant depression. The dilemma for many asylum-seeking parents is that many have fled their country of origin motivated to protect their children, only to find themselves in a detention environment. The capacity of parents to manage their own trauma and distress is of primary importance on mediating the effects of traumatizing or depriving environments on infants and young children. The traumatized parent may find it difficult to provide a "buffer" or protective function for their child if they are overwhelmed by their own experiences.

For many parents in immigration detention experiences of depression and guilt are common. Rates of depression, anxiety, trauma-related and physical symptoms increase with the length of time spent in detention (Green & Eagar, 2010). Witnessing the deterioration of a parent's mental functioning may have particularly negative impact on children as described in observational studies to have high rates of regressed behaviors, anxiety and attachment difficulties (Mares, Newman, & Dudley, 2002). Over 80% of adult detainees have been found to meet diagnostic criteria for depression and related mental disorders (Steel et al., 2004) suggesting that the impact on their children will be major. Mares and Jureidini (2004) report on a diagnostic survey of asylum seeker children in Australia and found that all 10 children aged 5 to 7 years had cognitive delay and that all children aged 7–17 years met diagnostic criteria for posttraumatic stress disorder and major depression with suicidal ideation. Significantly all these children had experienced further trauma while in the detention environment and were witness to riots, behavioral disturbance, and self-harm.

VULNERABILITY, RISK, AND PROTECTION

Child asylum seekers are particularly vulnerable to the impact of trauma. The outcome for these children reflects the impact of premigration trauma, the detention experience and the response of adult caregivers. Parenting and child protection are fundamentally compromised in traumatic environments (Newman & Steel, 2008).

Two particularly vulnerable groups of child asylum seekers are those born in detention and those unaccompanied minors seeking asylum having arrived alone. Infants have clear neurodevelopmental vulnerability and sensitivity to disruption of caretaking relationships and emotional interaction. Reports of pregnant asylum seekers in the United Kingdom describe women with anxiety during their pregnancy, later concerns about infant development and lack of confidence in themselves as parents. Women described feelings of guilt and shame at having an infant in detention and were concerned that their infant would be psychologically damaged (Mcleish, Cutler, & Stamer, 2002).

Unaccompanied children and adolescents experience not only the trauma of forced migration but the the burden of responsibility for the continuity and survival of their family and culture. In addition they are separated from parents or adult caregivers and significant numbers are orphaned. These children may have been directly targeted in their home countries and involved in war conflict and forced labor. The risks for unprotected child asylum seekers in terms of sexual exploitation and trafficking are significant. Identification of unaccompanied and separate children remains problematic and children may not have appropriate explanations or legal support in the process of seeking asylum (Bhabha, Crock, & Finch, 2006). Failure to recognize child-specific persecution (such as sexual abuse and forced marriage and female genital mutilation), results in underresponse to trauma and increases the risks of ongoing psychological disorder. A major issue within detention settings is the lack of child specialist mental health expertise and limited capacity to recognize signs of trauma or distress in children.

Extreme stress in child asylum seekers has been described as contributing to a severe withdrawal resulting in children feeling utterly helpless in their situation, frequently with overwhelmed parents (Bodegard, 2005). These children present with withdrawal, mutism and refusal to eat or drink requiring hospitalization. A highly publicized case in Australia raised significant concerns about the need to protect children even in the face of the impact of immigration law.

The case of S.B., an Iranian child held in detention with his family, initially in Woomera and then Villawood detention center in metropolitan Sydney, received extensive publicity and put the issue of child detention on the public agenda (Moorehead, 2006). S.B., aged five years, spent a period of 11 months in the Woomera detention facility in a remote Australian desert and was exposed to riots, self-harm, suicidal behavior, and violence. He became progressively more withdrawn and anxious, had nightmares, and started bedwetting. The family was transferred to Villawood detention center in Sydney, where the child was again exposed to behavioral disturbance and self-harm. He witnessed a significant suicide attempt and became progressively more withdrawn and mute. His condition deteriorated to the point that he refused to eat or drink, and he was admitted to the hospital on several occasions for dehydration. He showed some improvement each time he was admitted to the hospital but relapsed each time he was returned to detention. Several child psychiatrists and other professionals advised that S.B. should not be returned to detention and urged that he be released into the community along with his mother. This advice was neglected by the then Minister for Immigration, who argued that to do so would set a precedent for the release of other children. S.B.'s condition continued to deteriorate, and after six months in Villawood he was removed from his family, again against professional advice, and placed in a community foster care. His mother was released four months later, and his father eight months after that, when he was found to be a genuine refugee and granted a residency visa. At 12 years of age, S.B. remained under psychiatric care and had ongoing features of posttraumatic stress disorder, depression, and adjustment difficulties.

PROTECTING CHILD ASYLUM SEEKERS

Several United Nations committees and international nongovernment organizations have reported on the negative impact of immigration detention and particularly the mental health and developmental consequences. All reports have found that the prolonged detention of vulnerable groups is damaging to mental health and is directly related to the high prevalence of mental disorders found in these groups (see HREOC report). Community concern and advocacy on behalf of child asylum seekers in Australia, and increasing concerns about mental health issues in detention centers, gave impetus to some reforms in detention operations and a stated policy of avoiding the detention of children and families. In practice, the policy of off-shore (Christmas Island) housing of asylum seekers has negated this positive initiative.

The need to protect children and prevent mental health problems has created a complex situation where advocacy is a central component of the clinician's role and this may bring clinicians into conflict with government policy (Newman, Dudley, & Steel, 2008). In Australia there has been a discussion about the primacy of immigration law over child protection concerns and an ongoing need to advocate for the removal of children and their attachment figures from remote facilities. For clinicians significant ethical dilemmas present themselves—to work within or outside detention centers; how to treat when the environment and operations of detention are contributing in a major way to the disorders; and whether to engage in a highly politicized arena. Many child mental health clinicians are familiar with the need to advocate for children and their services, but not many have needed to learn the skills necessary to engage in a political process. Detained asylum seekers will inevitably experience some level of distress related to their situation and will deteriorate in situations of prolonged detention. Psychiatrists and mental health professionals have limited capacity to treat in this situation, but arguably have a greater role in raising concerns and awareness about a situation where human rights are violated (Dudley & Gale, 2002).

CONCLUSIONS: TRAUMA AND RECOVERY

Trauma on a massive scale, such as that experienced by many asylum seekers, raises challenges for traditional (Western) psychological models of adaptation and recovery. The term *trauma* in psychological theory usually describes individual internal responses. For asylum seekers trauma has been a collective experience and it often has a long history. Trauma of this type may involve multiple issues and threats to culture and meaning (Miller & Rasco, 2004). Responding to the individual's distress remains important but the cultural, political and historical meaning provide the context. In these situations, the survival of the child asylum seeker comes to symbolize the future continuity of the community and culture. The risks asylum seekers take to provide a future for their children are considerable.

Recovery from trauma and humanitarian crisis as described by Silove and Steel (1999), involves an involved process of reestablishing safety, security, and relationships. For children provision of and connection with attachment figures and consistent care is central to processing of trauma. Supporting parents in regaining a sense of parenting competence will also be important.

In the longer term, child asylum seekers need support to piece together a narrative account of their history of flight and resettlement, and to come to terms with the many losses they and their family have experienced.

Clinicians have a central role in this process, but also in advocating for the rights and welfare of children trapped within systems of deterrence and inappropriate detention.

REFERENCES

Bhabha, J., Crock, M., & Finch, N. (2006). *Seeking asylum alone: Unaccompa nied and separated children and refugee protection in Australia, the UK and the US.* Sydney: Federation Press.

Bodegard, G. (2005). Pervasive loss of function in asylum-seeking children in Sweden. *Acta Paediatrica, 94*, 1706–1707.

Dudley, M., & Gale, F. (2002). Psychiatrists as a moral community? Psychiatry under the Nazis and its contemporary relevance. *Australian and New Zealand Journal of Psychiatry, 36*, 585–594.

Green, J. P., & Eagar, K. (2010). The health of people in Australian immigration detention centres. *Medical Journal of Australia, 192*(2), 65–70.

Mares, S., & Jureidini, J. (2004). Psychiatric assessment of children and fami- lies in immigration detention. *Australia and New Zealand Journal of Public Health, 28*(6), 16–22.

Mares, S., Newman, L. K., & Dudley, M. (2002). Seeking refuge, losing hope: Par- ents and children in immigration detention. *Australasian Psychiatry, 10*, 91–96.

Mcleish, J., Cutler, S., & Stamer, C. (2002). *A crying shame: Pregnant asylum seekers and their babies in detention.* Retrieved from http://www.asylumsup- port.info/

Miller, K. E., & Rasco, L. M. (Eds.). (2004). *The mental health of refugees: Ecological approaches to healing and adaptation.* Mahwah, NJ: Lawrence Erlbaum Associates.

Moorehead, C. (2006). *Human cargo: A journey amongst refugees.* London: Vintage.

Murthy, R. S., & Lakshminarayana, R. (2006). Mental health consequences of war: A brief review of research findings. *World Psychiatry, 5*, 25–30.

Newman, L. K. (2009). *Harming children: Child asylum seekers in Australia.* Retrieved from http://www.org.au/refugees

Newman, L. K., Dudley, M., & Steel, Z. (2008). Asylum, detention and mental health in Australia. *Refugee Survey Quarterly, 27*(3), 111–127.

Newman, L. K., & Steel, Z. (2008). The child asylum seeker: Psychological and developmental impact of immigration detention. *Child and Adolescent Psychi- atric Clinic of North America, 17*, 665–687.

Silove, D., Austin, P., & Steel, Z. (2007). No refuge from terror: The impact of detention on the mental health and trauma affected refugees seeking asylum in Australia. *Transcultural Psychiatry, 44*, 359–393.

Silove, D., & Steel, Z. (1999). The psychosocial effects of torture, mass human rights violations and refugee trauma. *Journal of Nervous and Mental Disease, 107*, 200–207.

Silove, D., Steel, Z., & Walters, C. (2000). Policies of deterrence and the mental health of asylum seekers in Western countries. *Journal of the Australian Medical Association, 284*, 604–611.

Steel, Z., Momartin, S., Bateman, C., Hafshejani, A., Silove, D., Everson, N., Roy, K., Dudley, M., Newman, L., Blick, B., Mares, S. (2004). Psychiatric status of asylum seeker families held over a protected period in a remote detention centre in Australia. *Australian and New Zealand Journal of Public Health, 28*, 527–546.

UNHCR. (2000). *The state of the world's refugees: Fifty years of humanitarian intervention.* Oxford: Oxford University Press.

INDEX

abuse and, 156. *See also* Infant depression; Infant withdrawal; Maternal depression; Postnatal depression in developing countries; Prenatal depression in developing countries

Developmental sensitivity, early years, 35

Diagnostic and Statistical Manual (DSM-IV), early diagnosis of depression, 112

Diarrhea in children, postnatal depression and, 98, 99, 101, 102

Diffusion tensor imaging (DTI), 164

Disabilities, South African children, 41

Dismissing attachment, 140

Disorganized attachment, 134–35, 170

Displaced persons, 217, 221. *See also* Asylum seekers

Distal factors, 167

Diurnal rhythms, 181–82

Domestic violence: in families of street children, 13; in South Africa, 41–42, 51, 53–54

Dopamine, 113, 139, 164

Dose-response effect, 158

DRD4 alleles, 113, 121

Drug abuse. *See* Substance abuse

DTI. *See* Diffusion tensor imaging

Dual process model, 139

Dyadic states of consciousness, 115

Dysthymic disorder, sleep disturbances and, 190

Early attachment, 199–200; developmental pathways involved in borderline personality disorder (BPD) and, 140–45; experiences, stress regulation, mentalization, and borderline personality disorder (BPD) and, 135–38; individual differences in stress responsivity and, 139–40; origin of mentalization and, 130–31; quality of and early mentalization, 132–35; resilience in borderline personality disorder (BPD) and, 145–46

Early childhood development (ECD), 35

Early childhood development (ECD) in South Africa, 35–63; Apartheid Mental Health Act (2006), 36; background, 35–37; Child and Adolescent

Mental Health guidelines (2003), 36; child maltreatment prevention, 51, 53–54; Children's Act (2007), 36; defined, 37; disability and psychiatric disorders, 41; early childhood cognitive development before school years, 54–57; early education, 42–44; five NGOs area-based strategies, 56–57; hunger and nutrition, 40–41; impact of HIV/AIDS, 39–41, 47–51; income distribution and poverty, 39; interventions, 36–37, 44–45; morbidity and mortality, 39–40; National Integrated Plan for Early Childhood Development (NIP for ECD), 36–37; population and, 38; rehabilitation of malnourished children, 45–46; risk of maltreatment, 41–42

Early life stress (ELS): long-term consequences of, 197–98; natural experiments in the study of, 198–200. *See also* Child evacuations in the Helsinki Birth Cohort Study (HBCS)

Eastern Europe, HIV/AIDS in, 100

Eating disorders, 136

ECA-N, 121

ECD. *See* Early childhood development

EDEN study, 120

Edinburgh Postnatal Depression Scale (EPDS), 93, 116

Education: dropping out of school, 11, 14; early education in South Africa, 42–44, 54–57; *Libreta* (formal document that verifies school record), 14; transitioning off the streets and, 4, 18, 23, 28–29, 31. *See also* Early childhood development in South Africa; School experiences

El Alto slum of La Paz, Bolivia, 11. *See also* Transitioning off the streets in La Paz, Bolivia

ELS. *See* Early life stress

Emotional abuse, 141

Emotional development, postnatal depression and, 99–100

Emotional systems, in mammalians, 113

Empathy, 169

Endophenotypes, 113–14, 121

Environmental factors, sleep disturbances and, 182–88

EPDS. *See* Edinburgh Postnatal Depression Scale

Esperanza Program: background of, 6–7; elements of, 6; framework for success of, 24–27; Hogar Illimani (Illimani Home), 9; Hogar Sajama (Sajama Home), 9; perceptions and influence of, 19–24; permanent homes with a family model, 7; street outreach program, 6, 11; successful transitioning parameters, 6; transition homes, 6–7. *See also* Transitioning off the streets of La Paz, Bolivia

Ethiopia, postnatal depression in, 92, 97

Ethnicity, infant withdrawal and, 119, 120

Evidence-based interventions, for children with fetal alcohol spectrum syndrome (FASS), 156, 172

Experimental desynchronization setting, 115

Experimental sleep restriction studies, 182, 189

Exploitation, street children and, 2

Externalization, 136, 163

Extracurricular activities, for transitioning street youth, 6

Facial features, of children exposed to alcohol prenatally, 158, 160

Failure to thrive (FTT), 114

False beliefs, 130, 133

Families: homeless youth and, 4, 9, 11–13, 27, 28, 30, 31. *See also* Domestic violence; Mental health impacts of HIV/AIDS

FAS. *See* Fetal alcohol syndrome

FASD. *See* Fetal alcohol spectrum disorders

Fathers, infant-father attachment, 132

Faux pas tasks, 130

Fearful attachment, 140

Female genital mutilation, 220

Fetal alcohol spectrum disorders (FASD), 155, 158, 172

Fetal alcohol syndrome (FAS), 155, 158

Fight-flight-freeze, 139

Fighting defense, 114

Finland: child evacuations in the Helsinki Birth Cohort Study (HBCS), 199–211; register study of children placed out of the home due to Tuberculosis, 198–99

Finnish Causes of Death Register (CDR), 203

Finnish Hospital Discharge Register (HDR), 203

Focus groups, for street boys of La Paz, Bolivia, 7–8

Forced marriage, 220

Foster care, 156, 158, 163, 173, 198

Freezing defense, 114

FTT. *See* Failure to thrive

Future focus/orientation, of youth transitioning off the streets, 3, 24, 26, 29–30, 31

Gambia, postnatal depression in, 92

Gender differences: infant withdrawal and, 117, 119; prenatally drug exposed children, 164

Gender inequalities, postnatal depression and, 93–94, 98

Gene-environment correlation (rGE), 188

Gene-environment interactions (G X E), 188

General Household Survey 2008 (Statistics South Africa), 43

Genetics, 197; attachment disorders and, 113–14; mentalization and, 137–38; sleep and, 180–82, 184, 186, 187–88

Germany, detention of asylum seekers, 218

Gestation, depression in mothers and fetuses, 115–16

Gestational sleep, 180–81

Gini coefficient, 39

Global Strategy on Infant and Young Child Feeding, 98

"Godparent" program, 23

Grounded imagination, 135

Grounded theory approach, 8–9

Group counseling, for youth transitioning off the streets, 21–22

Growth impairment, 95–98

Growth indices, 95

Guyana, postnatal depression in, 92

ABOUT THE EDITORS AND CONTRIBUTORS

CATHERINE AYOUB holds an EdD in counseling and consulting psychology from Harvard University and a master's degree in psychiatric mental health nursing from Emory University. Currently she is director of research and evaluation at the Brazelton Touchpoints Center at Children's Hospital Boston, director of research at the Children and the Law Program at Massachusetts General Hospital, and an associate professor in psychology at Harvard Medical School. Her research and practice interests focus on the consequences of risk and trauma on child development and on the design and implementation of prevention and intervention systems to combat risk and promote resilience, with an emphasis on young children, families, and communities. Raised in Mexico, Dr. Ayoub has special expertise in clinical work and research with Latino families and in intervention programming in Central and South America.

LINDA BIERSTEKER is a psychologist and specialist in the field of early child development. She is research director at the Early Learning Resource Unit in Cape Town, South Africa. Her research has focused on policy development, programming, and training strategies for the early childhood development sector as well as on indicators and results-based monitoring and evaluation.

MARK E. BOYES received his PhD in psychology in 2010 from the University of Western Australia. His doctoral research focused on individual differences in stress reactivity and coping in the context of stressful situations. Dr. Boyes is a postdoctoral research officer in the Department of Social Policy and Intervention at the University of Oxford and is a junior research fellow at Wolfson College. He is currently working on the Young Carers project (http://www.youngcarers.org.za/), which is exploring the impact of living in an AIDS-affected family on children's mental and physical health, social development, and educational outcomes.

LUCIE CLUVER is a university lecturer at the University of Oxford's Department of Social Policy and Intervention and at the University of Cape Town's Department of Psychiatry and Mental Health. She trained as a social worker and has practiced in South Africa and the United Kingdom. Dr. Cluver works closely with the South African government to develop a strong evidence base for policy on AIDS-affected children and is a scientific advisor to the National Action Committee for Children Affected by AIDS. She speaks isiXhosa with a terrible accent and has a bad habit of missing flights.

PETER J. COOPER completed his doctorate and clinical training in Oxford, after which he held the University Lectureship in Psychopathology in Cambridge. Currently he is a research professor in psychopathology at the University of Reading, where, jointly with Lynne Murray, he runs the Winnicott Research Unit. He has been engaged for many years in research on the nature and treatment of postpartum depression, including research on maternal mood disorder and child development in Africa. A further strand to Peter Cooper's collaborative work with Lynne Murray concerns the intergenerational transmission of anxiety disorders. A major aspect of this work is the systematic investigation of novel treatments for child anxiety disorder.

ANDREW DAWES is an Emeritus Professor in Psychology at the University of Cape Town, an associate fellow in social policy and social work at the University of Oxford, and a fellow of the Association of Psychological Science. His research seeks to produce evidence to inform social policy directed at improving the situation of young children living in poverty in South Africa.

HIRAM E. FITZGERALD is associate provost for university outreach and engagement and university distinguished professor of psychology at Michigan State University. He is president of the National Outreach Scholarship Conference. Dr. Fitzgerald's research includes the study of infant and family development in a community context, the impact of fathers on early child development, the implementation of systemic models of organizational process and change, the etiology of alcoholism and coactive psychopathology, the digital divide and the youth–computer interface, and broad issues related to the scholarship of engagement and engaged scholarship. He has received numerous awards, including the ZERO TO THREE Dolley Madison Award for Outstanding Lifetime Contributions to the Development and Well Being of Very Young Children and the World Association for Infant Mental Health's designation as Honorary President.

PETER FONAGY is Freud Memorial Professor of Psychoanalysis and head of the Research Department of Clinical, Educational, and Health Psychology at University College London. He is chief executive at the Anna Freud Centre in London. He is a clinical psychologist and a training and supervising analyst in the British Psycho-Analytical Society in child and adult analysis. He holds a number of important positions, which include chairing the Postgraduate Centre of the International Psychoanalytic Association and a fellowship in the British Academy. His clinical interests center around issues of borderline psychopathology, violence, and early attachment relationships. His work attempts to integrate empirical research with psychoanalytic theory.

FRANCES GARDNER is professor of child and family psychology in the Department of Social Policy and Intervention University of Oxford, and fellow of Wolfson College. She is codirector of the Centre for Evidence-Based Intervention and was the first director of the graduate program in evidence-based social intervention at Oxford. Her research focuses on risk factors in the development of psychological problems in young people, especially family and parenting factors. She has conducted several randomized controlled trials of community-based parenting programs in the United Kingdom and United States as well as systematic reviews of family interventions. Her longitudinal studies include one that investigates factors promoting resilience in orphans and vulnerable children in South Africa. She serves on the Scientific Advisory Board for the U.K. National Academy of Parenting Practitioners, for SFI, and for the Danish National Centre for Social Research and on a UNODC Expert Panel on worldwide family skills training.

ANTOINE GUEDENEY was named full professor of child and adolescent psychiatry in 2000 at the University of Paris Denis Diderot. He is the head of the Department of Child and Adolescent Psychiatry at the Paris Bichat-Claude Bernard Hospital, APHP, and is a member of the INSERM U 669 research unit. He is the current president of the World Association for Infant Mental Health (2008–2012). He has been the editor of the journal *Devenir* since 1989. His research has focused on early depression and social withdrawal behavior in infancy, on attachment, and on early prevention in infancy.

KRISTIN HUANG completed her doctorate in human development and psychology at the Harvard Graduate School of Education in 2008. She is currently the executive director of Kaya Children International, where she is engaged in program development and research related to the unique needs of children on the streets, primarily in Latin America. Her research is focused on understanding risk and resilience in street children, effective therapeutic interventions, children's school experiences, and factors associated with dropout.

PATRICK LUYTEN is assistant professor and codirector of the Psychoanalysis Unit at the Department of Psychology, University of Leuven (Belgium). Dr. Luyten's main research interest focuses on the role of personality, stress, and interpersonal processes in depression, chronic fatigue syndrome, and fibromyalgia. He is currently also involved in studies on mentalization-based treatment of patients with borderline personality disorder. He is a visiting professor at the Research Department of Clinical, Educational, and Health Psychology, University College London, and adjunct assistant professor at the Yale Child Study Center, New Haven, Connecticut.

VIBEKE MOE received her PhD in developmental psychology in 2002 from the University of Oslo. She is a specialist in clinical psychology and is currently working as a senior researcher at the National Network for Infant Mental Health of the Centre for Child and Adolescent Mental Health in Norway. Her research and clinical work has focused on children at risk, parental substance abuse and psychiatric problems, early affective development, mother–infant interaction and father–infant interaction, and early intervention.

LOUISE NEWMAN is professor of developmental psychiatry at Monash University, Melbourne, Australia, and director of the Centre for Developmental Psychology and Psychiatry. She is an infant psychiatrist and undertakes research in the area of early trauma and parenting disturbances. She is chair of the Detention Expert Health Advisory Group advising the Australian government on the health needs of asylum seekers.

DON OPERARIO received his PhD in social psychology in 1998 from the University of Massachusetts at Amherst. He completed an National Institute of Mental Health postdoctoral fellowship in health psychology and behavioral medicine at the University of California, San Francisco.

Currently he is associate professor of medical sciences in the Program in Public Health at Brown University. His research has focused on HIV prevention in vulnerable populations and the consequences of HIV/AIDS on families and communities.

E. JUULIA PAAVONEN received her MD degree in 2000 from the University of Helsinki. In 2003, she received her BSocSc degree in statistics from the University of Helsinki. In 2005, she received a PhD degree in child psychiatry from the University of Helsinki. In 2010, she became adjunct professor in neuropsychiatric epidemiology at the University of Helsinki. Currently she works as a senior researcher at the National Institute for Health and Welfare. Her research has focused on epidemiological risk factors for children's mental health and behavior, particularly sleeping difficulties and chronic sleep restriction, as well as on parental mental health problems and their impact on children.

CHRISTINE E. PARSONS received her PhD in child psychology in 2008 from the National University of Ireland, Maynooth. She is currently a postdoctoral researcher at the Department of Psychiatry, University of Oxford. Her research focuses on the biological basis of the evolving parent–infant relationship and examines factors that might compromise this relationship.

CAMPBELL PAUL is a consultant infant and child psychiatrist at the Royal Children's Hospital, Melbourne, and Honorary Principal Fellow in the Department of Psychiatry at the University of Melbourne. At the university, he and colleagues have established a graduate diploma and a master's course in infant and parent mental health. This course developed out of his long-standing experience in pediatric consultation liaison psychiatry and work in infant parent psychotherapy. He has a special interest in the understanding of the inner world of the baby, particularly as it informs therapeutic work with infants and their parents. He is a member of the Board of Directors of the World Association for Infant Mental Health and has been a participant in and organizer of a number of local and international conferences and activities in the field of infant mental health. He is also a consultant psychiatrist at the Victorian Aboriginal Health Service and has also been involved in the establishment of the Koori Kids Mental Health Network.

ANU-KATRIINA PESONEN received her PhD in developmental psychology in 2004 from the University of Helsinki. Currently she is senior lecturer in clinical child psychology at the Institute of Behavioral Sciences at the University of Helsinki. In addition to studying the programming effects of early life stress, her research has focused on the development outcomes of children born severely premature, children's sleep, and temperamental development. A specific study interest are the developmental correlates of the HPA axis function and stress physiology in children and adults.

KAIJA PUURA received her MD in 1985 and her PhD in child psychiatry in 1998 from the University of Tampere. Currently she is adjunct professor in child psychiatry at the University of Tampere and assistant chief of child psychiatry at the Tampere University Hospital. Her research has focused on parent–infant interaction in infancy and on assessment and interventions for infants and families in primary services.

KATRI RÄIKKÖNEN received her PhD in psychology in 1990 from the University of Helsinki. Currently she is the professor of developmental, personality, and clinical psychology at the University of Helsinki and director of the National Graduate Program of Psychology in Finland. Her research has focused on early life origins, including fetal programming and early life stress; on psychological development; and on mental health over the life course.

OUTI SAARENPÄÄ-HEIKKILÄ received her MD from the Medical School of Tampere University, Finland, in 1984. She received specialty certification as a pediatrician in 1991 and in pediatric neurology in 1997, from the same university. The topic of her thesis (2001) is daytime sleepiness in schoolchildren. Sleep medicine is still the focus of her research. Currently she is a consultant in pediatric neurology in the Pediatric Clinic of Tampere University Hospital.

TORILL SIQVELAND is a psychologist. She is currently a doctoral student in the Department of Psychology, University of Oslo, and at the National Network for Infant Mental Health in Norway. Her research is focused on children born of mothers with substance abuse and psychiatric problems.

KARI SLINNING received her PhD in developmental psychology in 2004 from the University of Oslo. Currently she is working as a child psychologist and senior researcher at the National Network for Infant Mental Health in Norway and at the Division of Mental Health of the National Institute of Public Health. Her clinical work and research have focused on children living with families with substance abuse and perinatal depression.

ALAN STEIN is professor of child and adolescent psychiatry at the University of Oxford. He is South African and received his medical training at the University of Witwatersrand. Most of his postgraduate medical training was undertaken at Oxford. He has held joint senior research fellowships at the University of Oxford and the University of Cambridge and was subsequently professor of child and adolescent mental health at the Royal Free and University College Medical School and Tavistock Centre. He is also an honorary fellow of the Child, Youth, Family, and Social Development Program of the HSRC in South Africa. His main area of research concerns the development of young children in the face of adversity. These potential adversities include parental physical illness (HIV and cancer); psychological disorders, including depression, anxiety, and eating disorders; and poverty and malnutrition. The ultimate aim of this work is to develop interventions to enhance children's early development and support their families.

LANE STRATHEARN is an assistant professor in the departments of Pediatrics and Psychiatry at Baylor College of Medicine and a developmental pediatrician at Texas Children's Hospital, Houston. His research and clinical work focus on maternal neglect and the neurobiology of mother–infant attachment, which was also the topic of his dissertation for his recently obtained PhD in medicine from the University of Queensland, Australia. He has studied the long-term effects of child maltreatment on cognitive and emotional development as well as early childhood factors that may help to protect against abuse or neglect. His most recent National Institutes of Health grants will support research into maternal brain responses of cocaine-addicted mothers and the potential role of intranasal oxytocin to enhance maternal caregiving.

MARK TOMLINSON received his PhD in developmental psychology in 2004 from the University of Reading, United Kingdom. Currently he is associate professor in the Department of Psychology at Stellenbosch University, South Africa. His research has focused on postpartum depression; parent–infant interaction; infant and child development; research priority-setting processes; the development of community-based interventions for parent–infant interaction; and behavioral interventions in the areas of HIV, mother–child transmission of HIV, neonatal illness, and reducing alcohol use during the perinatal period.

KATHERINE S. YOUNG is currently studying for her DPhil in child and adolescent psychiatry at the University of Oxford. Her research focuses on the effects of postnatal depression on the functional neuroanatomy of adult responsivity to infant cues.

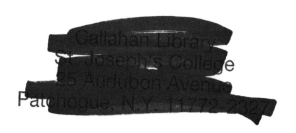